Injectables and Nonsurgical Rejuvenation

Editor

JESSYKA G. LIGHTHALL

FACIAL PLASTIC SURGERY CLINICS OF NORTH AMERICA

www.facialplastic.theclinics.com

Consulting Editor
J. REGAN THOMAS

August 2022 • Volume 30 • Number 3

ELSEVIER

1600 John F. Kennedy Boulevard • Suite 1800 • Philadelphia, Pennsylvania, 19103-2899

http://www.theclinics.com

FACIAL PLASTIC SURGERY CLINICS OF NORTH AMERICA Volume 30, Number 3
August 2022 ISSN 1064-7406, ISBN-13: 978-0-323-85005-6

Editor: Stacy Eastman
Developmental Editor: Ann Gielou M. Posedio

Facial Plastic Surgery Clinics of North America (ISSN 1064-7406) is published quarterly by Elsevier Inc., 360 Park Avenue South, New York, NY 10010-1710. Months of issue are February, May, August, and November. Business and Editorial Offices: 1600 John F. Kennedy Blvd., Suite 1800, Philadelphia, PA 19103-2899. Periodicals postage paid at New York, NY, and additional mailing offices. Subscription prices are $420.00 per year (US individuals), $922.00 per year (US institutions), $468.00 per year (Canadian individuals), $950.00 per year (Canadian institutions), $557.00 per year (foreign individuals), $950.00 per year (foreign institutions), $100.00 per year (US students), $100.00 per year (Canadian students), and $255.00 per year (foreign students). Foreign air speed delivery is included in all *Clinics* subscription prices. All prices are subject to change without notice. POSTMASTER: Send address changes to *Facial Plastic Surgery Clinics*, Elsevier Health Sciences Division, Subscription Customer Service, 3251 Riverport Lane, Maryland Heights, MO 63043. **Customer service: 1-800-654-2452 (US and Canada); 1-314-447-8871 (outside US and Canada); Fax: 314-447-8029; E-mail: journalscustomerservice-usa@elsevier.com (for print support); journalsonlinesupport-usa@elsevier.com (for online support).**

Reprints. For copies of 100 or more of articles in this publication, please contact the Commercial Reprints Department, Elsevier Inc., 360 Park Avenue South, New York, NY 10010-1710. Tel.: 212-633-3874; Fax: 212-633-3820; E-mail: reprints@elsevier.com.

Facial Plastic Surgery Clinics of North America is covered in *MEDLINE/PubMed* (*Index Medicus*).

Contributors

CONSULTING EDITOR

J. REGAN THOMAS, MD
Professor, Facial Plastic and Reconstructive
Surgery, Department of Otolaryngology–Head
and Neck Surgery, Northwestern University
Feinberg School of Medicine, Chicago, Illinois

EDITOR

JESSYKA G. LIGHTHALL, MD, FACS
Chief, Division of Facial Plastic and
Reconstructive Surgery, Medical Director,
Esteem Penn State Health Cosmetic
Associates, Associate Professor, Department
of Otolaryngology–Head and Neck Surgery,
Director, Facial Nerve Disorders Clinic, Penn
State College of Medicine, Penn State Hershey
Medical Center, Hershey, Pennsylvania

AUTHORS

KATHERINE BERRY, MD
Assistant Professor, Department of
Dermatology, Penn State Health Hershey
Medical Center, Hershey, Pennsylvania

JASON D. BLOOM, MD, FACS
Bloom Facial Plastic Surgery, Bryn Mawr,
Pennsylvania

PAUL J. CARNIOL, MD
Clinical Professor, Facial Plastic Surgery,
Department of Otolaryngology–Head and Neck
Surgery, Rutgers New Jersey Medical School,
Newark, New Jersey

TODD V. CARTEE, MD
Associate Professor, Department of
Dermatology, Milton S. Hershey Medical
Center, Hershey, Pennsylvania

JOHN J. CHI, MD, MPHS
Division of Facial Plastic and Reconstructive
Surgery, Washington University Facial Plastic
Surgery Center, Washington University in

St. Louis School of Medicine, Creve Coeur,
Missouri

KENNEDY DIERKS
Research Assistant, Carniol Plastic Surgery,
Summit, New Jersey; Student, Joint
Bachelor's/M.D. Program, Seton Hall
University, South Orange, New Jersey

YADRO DUCIC, MD
Dallas, Texas

FRED G. FEDOK, MD, FACS
The Fedok Plastic Surgery and Laser Center,
Foley, Alabama

KATHERINE HALLOCK, MD
Assistant Professor, Department of
Dermatology, Penn State Health Hershey
Medical Center, Hershey, Pennsylvania

JOANNA KAM, MD
Georgia Center for Facial Plastic Surgery,
Evans, Georgia

KIAN KARIMI, MD
Facial Plastic and Reconstructive Surgery,
Medical Director and Founder, Rejuva Medical
Aesthetics, Los Angeles, California

AMIT KOCHHAR, MD
Facial Plastic and Reconstructive Surgery,
Pacific Neuroscience Institute, Los Angeles,
California

THEDA KONTIS, MD
Associate Professor, Department of
Otolaryngology-Head and Neck Surgery,
Department of Plastic and Reconstructive
Surgery, Johns Hopkins, Baltimore,
Maryland

PARVESH KUMAR, BA
Pacific Neuroscience Institute, Los Angeles,
California

CHARLENE LAM, MD, MPH
Associate Professor, Department of
Dermatology, Penn State Health Hershey
Medical Center, Hershey, Pennsylvania

JESSYKA G. LIGHTHALL, MD, FACS
Chief, Division of Facial Plastic and
Reconstructive Surgery, Medical Director,
Esteem Penn State Health Cosmetic
Associates, Associate Professor, Department
of Otolaryngology–Head and Neck Surgery,
Director, Facial Nerve Disorders Clinic,
Penn State College of Medicine, Penn State
Hershey Medical Center, Hershey,
Pennsylvania

MYRIAM LOYO, MD, MCR
Associate Professor, Division of Facial Plastic
and Reconstructive Surgery, Department of
Otolaryngology and Head and Neck Surgery,
Oregon Health & Sciences University, Portland,
Oregon

JEFFREY DESMOND MARKEY, MD
Facial Plastic Surgeon, Ascentist Plastic
Surgery, Leawood, Kansas

HILLARY A. NEWSOME, MD
Division of Facial Plastic and Reconstructive
Surgery, Washington University Facial Plastic
Surgery Center, Washington University in St.
Louis School of Medicine, Creve Coeur,
Missouri

KEON M. PARSA, MD
Department of Otolaryngology-Head and Neck
Surgery, MedStar Georgetown University
Hospital, Washington, DC

NOAH SAAD, MD
Fellow, Division of Plastic and Reconstructive
Surgery, Department of Surgery, Joe R.
and Teresa Lozano Long School of Medicine
UT Health San Antonio, San Antonio,
Texas

CHRISTEN B. SAMAAN, MD
Department of Dermatology, Milton S. Hershey
Medical Center, Hershey, Pennsylvania

JORDAN SAND, MD
Spokane Center for Facial Plastic Surgery,
Spokane, Washington

TOM SHOKRI, MD
Assistant Professor of Surgery, George
Washington University, Washington, DC

MICHAEL SOMENEK, MD
Somenek + Pittman MD, Washington, DC

EMILY A. SPATARO, MD
Assistant Professor, Division of Facial
Plastic and Reconstructive Surgery,
Department of Otolaryngology–Head and
Neck Surgery, Washington University in
St. Louis School of Medicine, St Louis,
Missouri

CHRISTIAN L. STALLWORTH, MD
Clinical Associate Professor, Director, Division
of Facial Plastic and Reconstructive Surgery,
Department of Otolaryngology–Head and
Neck Surgery, Joe R. and Teresa Lozano
Long School of Medicine, UT Health San
Antonio, Texas Plastic Surgery, San Antonio,
Texas

ANGELA STURM, MD, FACS
Private Practice, Bellaire, Texas; Assistant
Clinical Professor, Department of
Otolaryngology–Head and Neck Surgery,
University of Texas Medical Branch,
Galveston, Texas

SCOTT WALEN, MD
Division of Facial Plastic and Reconstructive
Surgery, Department of Otolaryngology–Head
and Neck Surgery, The Pennsylvania State

University, College of Medicine, Hershey, Pennsylvania

WILLIAM MATTHEW WHITE, MD
Facial Plastic Surgeon, Dr. Matthew White Facial Plastic Surgery, New York, New York

HARRY V. WRIGHT, MD, MS
Wright Spellman Plastic Surgery, Sarasota, Florida

GRACE T. WU, MD
Department of Otorhinolaryngology, University of Pennsylvania, Philadelphia, Pennsylvania

KASRA ZIAI, MD
Department of Otolaryngology–Head and Neck Surgery, The Pennsylvania State University, Milton S. Hershey Medical Center, Hershey, Pennsylvania

Contents

> Facial aging is a multifactorial process that occurs due to alterations in the skin, soft tissue, and bony skeleton. When considering treatments for the aging face and neck, a multifaceted approach targeting each of these areas should be considered. Although surgical intervention remains a key component to the holistic care of the aging face patient, a multitude of minimally invasive techniques is now available to optimize the care of the patient seeking rejuvenation. Proper patient evaluation and counseling on realistic expectations are critical and will be discussed here. A brief overview of common minimally invasive treatments will be presented.

> Photoaging is a complex process of skin changes associated with chronic ultraviolet exposure. Prevention with photoprotection and treatment with topical retinoids are the core components of a topical antiaging regimen. Other topicals such as hydroquinone, vitamin C, niacinamide, and alpha hydroxyl acid can be added based on specific concerns. However, caution must be used with some of these products as the stability and absorption are major considerations. A simple topical regimen will reduce irritability and enhance compliance.

> Hyaluronic acid (HA) is the most common dermal filler in use. It improves wrinkles and volume loss not only by filling and volumizing but also by hydrating the injected area with its water affinity. It is a naturally occurring component of skin, and there is a negligible risk of immunologic or allergic reaction with injection. It is rapidly degraded by the injection of hyaluronidase, thus creating an ideal injectable material that is low risk and reversible. Its duration of effect may be longer than expected based on bioavailability of the HA product due to collagen synthesis or fibroblast stimulation.

> Periorbital hyperpigmentation (POH) is a common aesthetic concern that impacts patients' emotional well-being and quality of life. POH can be difficult to manage as the etiology is often multifactorial or difficult to elucidate. An understanding of different contributing factors and ability to classify hyperpigmentation can aid in the management of POH. Classification of POH is divided into pigmented, vascular, structural, and mixed subtypes. A wide array of treatment options has

been proposed belying the challenges inherent to improving POH. Modalities vary from topical therapies, chemical peels, dermal fillers, and lasers, to surgical intervention. Because POH can be multifactorial, successful management of POH will depend on elucidating the etiology and often requires a combination of therapies.

Nonsurgical periocular rejuvenation presents varied options to the practitioner. The most common current inject modalities for rejuvenation include hyaluronic acid (HA), platelet-rich plasma (PRP), calcium hydroxyapatite, and poly-L-lactic acid. This article provides a summary of recent publications regarding each injectable as well as the description of pertinent periocular anatomy. The modern injector should possess an understanding of each modality for a safe and rejuvenated result.

This article reviews the evaluation and techniques for facial skin rejuvenation using the fractionated carbon dioxide laser. It includes a detailed overview of laser skin rejuvenation and discusses the potential complications associated with this procedure. A review of clinical outcomes in the literature is also included.

Injectable filler is one of the most common cosmetic procedures performed annually. An aging face shows a characteristic loss of volume in the deep fat pads of the midface. The goal of midfacial rejuvenation with injectable filler is to restore lost volume, with the suborbicularis fat pad and deep medial cheek fat being the most critical areas. Filler can be instilled here with a cannula or needle with successful outcomes. However, this procedure is not without complications if proper technique and underlying anatomy are not respected.

Soft tissue filler injections have become the second most common noninvasive cosmetic procedure performed in the United States, accounting for roughly 26% of all noninvasive procedures. As experience with filler injections has increased, so too have the applications and uses throughout the face. The popularity of "liquid," or nonsurgical, rhinoplasty has grown considerably with both patients and surgeons over the last decade. First documented in 2006, numerous descriptions of technique and application have grown in tandem with the increasing popularity of nonsurgical rhinoplasty procedures. Although nasal injections remain an "off-label" use in the United States, hyaluronic acid fillers have gained multiple applications for the nose. These include, but are not limited to, leveling a dorsal hump through the addition of volume above and below the dorsal convexity, filling of visible nasal concavities, correcting upper and middle third asymmetries, as well as improving the under-rotated or under the projected tip. Though attractive to both patient and surgeon for various reasons, nasal filler injections are not without risk, and knowledge of nasal surgical anatomy and management of complications are critical for safe, viable outcomes.

The lips are a central and essential feature of facial appearance and esthetics. When looking at attractive faces, we spend most of our time observing the eyes and lips, while the rest of the facial features fade away. Full lips are beautiful and youthful. Treatments to enhance the lips have long been pursued. In the 1990s, hyaluronic acid (HA) fillers revolutionized the market for facial esthetics. HA fillers' safety profile, quick recovery, and natural results have made it the preferred option for lip enhancement with or without complimentary neurotoxin. This article will discuss how to evaluate and treat the lip for enhancement using these techniques.

Cosmetic procedures to combat the effects of aging are increasing in demand. Surgical interventions, such as rhytidectomy, have long been the standard method of providing a more youthful appearance. However, these procedures are costly, often require general anesthesia, and have potential risks such as scarring and prolonged recovery. A safe, effective, alternative to surgery is the nonsurgical thread-lift. Nevertheless, proper patient selection is critical for optimal outcomes and for patient and provider satisfaction. Over the past decade, these treatments have gained significant popularity for patients to achieve a more rejuvenated appearance with less complications and minimal downtime.

Microneedling, also referred to as percutaneous collagen induction therapy, uses small needles to create mechanical injury to the skin, stimulating the wound-healing cascade and new collagen formation. Compared with other skin resurfacing techniques, microneedling preserves the epidermis and is nonablative, therefore reducing inflammation, downtime, and risk of dyspigmentation. In addition to increasing collagen production in fibroblasts, microneedling also helps normalize cell function of keratinocytes and melanocytes and can be used to increase absorption of topical medications, growth factors, or deliver radiofrequency directly to the dermis. The benefits of microneedling, associated procedures, indications for use, technical considerations, and potential complications are discussed.

As aging occurs, jawline definition is often lost. A thorough understanding of facial anatomy combined with a detailed evaluation of each patient's facial structure is key when addressing aesthetic concerns of the jawline. Several treatment modalities, including dermal fillers, neurotoxins, deoxycholic acid, and polydioxanone threads, can be used. A multifaceted approach can help optimize patient outcomes.

 Video content accompanies this article at http://www.facialplastic.theclinics.com

Nonsurgical skin tightening in the neck is an area of significant growth with seemingly countless devices. Optimal treatment choice depends on the patient's concerns, anatomy, and lifestyle. Patients with minimal skin laxity, but dynamic platysmal bands may benefit from botulinum toxin injections. Mild to moderately lax skin can be addressed with microfocused ultrasound or radiofrequency with microneedling. Significant sun damage and laxity can both be addressed with fractional ablative lasers. Options for submental preplatysmal fat include percutaneous radiofrequency, radiofrequency-helium plasma, deoxycholic acid injections, and cryolipolysis. Of these, percutaneous radiofrequency has the highest patient satisfaction and lowest complication rate.

Jordan Sand and Scott Walen

Both nonsurgical and surgical modalities for the treatment of hair loss are being used by providers at an increasing rate worldwide. Men and woman are affected by hair loss, but the pathophysiology of the hair loss is thought to be different between sexes; therefore, gender must play a role in treatment decisions. Currently, there are 3 Food and Drug Administration–approved nonsurgical androgenetic alopecia treatments: minoxidil, finasteride, and low-light laser therapy. Platelet-rich plasma injections are showing promise as a single modality and as an adjunct to other nonsurgical and surgical treatments of androgenetic alopecia.

FACIAL PLASTIC SURGERY CLINICS OF NORTH AMERICA

SERIES OF RELATED INTEREST

Clinics in Plastic Surgery
https://www.plasticsurgery.theclinics.com
Otolaryngologic Clinics
https://www.oto.theclinics.com
Dermatologic Clinics
https://www.derm.theclinics.com

THE CLINICS ARE AVAILABLE ONLINE!
Access your subscription at:
www.theclinics.com

Foreword
Injectables and Nonsurgical Rejuvenation

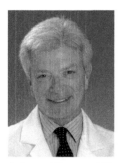

J. Regan Thomas, MD
Consulting Editor

In recent years, increasing interest in more minimally invasive treatments of facial appearance has continued to progress and grow. These treatments and procedures have simultaneously developed those interests in facial appearance enhancement in a broader age range of potential patients. No doubt the prevalence of various components of social media has also had a significant impact on the awareness of the public of these procedures and treatments as well as an enhanced self-evaluation and personal appearance goals. A greater desire for earlier facial appearance and antiaging treatments continues to grow as well as a desire for less-invasive procedures by more traditional age groups.

Facial plastic surgeons in this modern environment need to be aware of the various treatment options as they become available. Accordingly, they should have the knowledge and expertise to use these treatments optimally and with expert patient selection. Likewise, patients need to be educated and guided to make appropriate treatment selection decisions. As part of that process, the treating facial plastic surgeons, in addition to their treatment expertise and skills, must also make appropriate patient selections, decide on most useful modalities, and be prepared to educate their patients on options available to them, risks, and realistic outcomes.

As guest editor for this issue of *Facial Plastic Surgery Clinics of North America*, Dr Lighthall has organized an outstanding group of expert, experienced, and knowledgeable contributing authors. The authors provide an interesting and diversely wide array of treatment options, including techniques and technologies that can successfully improve and enhance the patient's facial appearance. The outcome of these contributions and expert discussions results in a unique source of useful and pragmatic information for these components of facial treatment. I appreciate the well-organized and resourceful contributions of this group of expert authors, and I am pleased to offer this collection of useful information through this issue to our readership.

J. Regan Thomas, MD
Facial Plastic and Reconstructive Surgery
Department of Otolaryngology
Head and Neck Surgery
Northwestern University School of Medicine
60 East Delaware Place
Chicago, IL 60611, USA

E-mail address:
regan.thomas@nm.org

Facial Plast Surg Clin N Am 30 (2022) xiii
https://doi.org/10.1016/j.fsc.2022.05.001
1064-7406/22/© 2022 Published by Elsevier Inc.

Preface

Injectables and Nonsurgical Rejuvenation of the Face and Neck

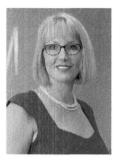

Jessyka G. Lighthall, MD, FACS
Editor

The practice of Facial Plastic and Reconstructive Surgery continues to expand and evolve. Recent surveys from the American Academy of Facial Plastic and Reconstructive Surgery as well as the American Society of Plastic Surgeons show continual increases in patients seeking minimally invasive treatments to address the aging face and neck. A cohort of younger of patients also present seeking "prejuvenation" procedures to minimize or delay the appearance of facial aging or to enhance their already youthful countenances. This has been compounded by the "selfie" era and "zoom dysmorphia" that exist in our current environment that may draw attention to real or perceived flaws.

Due to the complexity of facial aging affecting the skin, soft tissue, and bony skeleton, a multifaceted approach targeting each of these areas is often recommended for optimal rejuvenation. A plethora of technologies and techniques exists to combat each area of facial aging, and more are rapidly being developed to garner a corner of the minimally invasive aesthetic market. It may therefore be challenging to stay up-to-date on available technologies and techniques in the current environment.

In addition, with the social media boom, patients present having done "research" and often have misconceptions about what they want or need to treat their individual aging concerns. They may also have unrealistic expectations that a minimally invasive treatment may provide results similar to a more invasive surgical result. Aesthetic providers must have knowledge of the multitude of treatments available in order to help guide patients to a treatment plan that will provide the most natural rejuvenation. Often, this means reeducating patients regarding the aging process and modalities recommended for their specific circumstances with extensive counseling to establish a realistic expectation of outcomes.

Although surgery is still an essential component of facial and neck rejuvenation, this issue of *Facial Plastic Surgery Clinics of North America* is dedicated to discussing many of the commonly used minimally invasive therapies that may be used as primary or adjunctive procedures for facial and neck rejuvenation. This issue first discusses the aging process and reviews the evaluation and treatment planning of the aging face patient. Our experts then provide evidence-based reviews of medical-grade skin care, the use of injectible fillers, the treatment of periocular hypervascularity and pigmentation, resurfacing for skin rejuvenation, the use of threads for soft tissue lifting, adjuncts for hair rejuvenation, discussion of

Facial Plast Surg Clin N Am 30 (2022) xv–xvi
https://doi.org/10.1016/j.fsc.2022.03.001
1064-7406/22/© 2022 Published by Elsevier Inc.

technologies for soft tissue tightening and lipolysis, and review of the minimally invasive regional treatments of the face and neck.

I would like to thank all of the authors for providing their expertise in the fields of facial plastic surgery and dermatology. I hope that this issue helps readers develop a better understanding of the technologies and techniques available and to determine ideal patient selection, understand realistic outcomes and limitations of each therapy, and learn how to minimize complications to provide ultimate patient satisfaction. Although each article has a focus on a given treatment type or region, it cannot be overstated enough that more often than not optimal rejuvenation is obtained from an individualized and multimodal approach to aging.

Jessyka G. Lighthall, MD, FACS
Division of Facial Plastic &
Reconstructive Surgery
Esteem Penn State Health Cosmetic Associates
Department of Otolaryngology-Head & Neck
Surgery
Facial Nerve Disorders Clinic
Penn State College of Medicine
500 University Drive H-091
Hershey, PA 17033, USA

E-mail address:
jlighthall@pennstatehealth.psu.edu

Evaluation and Treatment Planning for the Aging Face Patient

Fred G. Fedok, MD[a], Jessyka G. Lighthall, MD[b],*

KEYWORDS

- Cosmetic evaluation • Cosmetic surgery • Facial plastic surgery • Aging face • Minimally invasive
- Facial rejuvenation • Patient evaluation

KEY POINTS

- Although surgery is still a mainstay of facial rejuvenation, a multitude of nonsurgical minimally invasive techniques exist for facial rejuvenation.
- Careful patient selection and counseling on realistic expectations is a critical component of the evaluation and treatment planning of the aging face patient.
- As facial aging is multifactorial, a multimodal approach to care provides optimal results.

INTRODUCTION

Facial aging is a multifactorial process that occurs due to alterations in the skin, soft tissue, and bony skeleton. When considering treatments for the aging face, a multifaceted approach targeting each of these areas should be considered. Although surgical intervention is a key component to the holistic care of the aging face patient, there is an expanding group of patients seeking nonsurgical esthetic interventions for rejuvenation with a nearly 175% increase in minimally invasive procedures in the past 20 years.[1] A plethora of minimally invasive procedures, technologies and techniques exist either as primary interventions or as adjuncts to surgery. It behooves one to have a firm understanding of the aging process and awareness of the available treatment options in order to provide optimal rejuvenation. In this article, we will provide an overview of the aging process, discuss the evaluation of the patient seeking facial aesthetic surgery, and provide a brief overview of minimally invasive techniques available for use in treatment planning. A more in-depth discussion of these techniques will be discussed in other chapters in this issue.

THE CHARACTERISTICS OF THE AGING FACE
The Skin

Both intrinsic and extrinsic factors are determinants of aging of the skin causing textural irregularities, pigmentation changes, prominent vasculature, and loss of tone with sagging (**Fig. 1**).[2,3] Intrinsic (or chronologic) aging is due to the passage of time and affects individuals at variable rates. This is genetically determined and tends to be familial in nature. Although aging progresses in a similar fashion for all, one will see characteristic differences in apparent skin aging between ethnicities, with people of darker skin color exhibiting less signs of intrinsic aging.[4] Overall there is general thinning of the dermis with a loss of elasticity and various degrees of skin sagging secondary to dermal relaxation and involution of various skin "ligaments" and other support mechanisms. There is a decrease in collagen and elastin synthesis and an increase in collagen fragmentation, primarily due to extrinsic factors.[5,6]

The most profound variable causing extrinsic (environmental) skin aging is ultraviolet radiation from sunlight although there are other important extrinsic factors including tobacco use, diet,

a The Fedok Plastic Surgery and Laser Center, 113 East Fern Avenue, Foley, AL 36535, USA; b Division of Facial Plastic and Reconstructive Surgery, Department of Otolaryngology-Head and Neck Surgery, Penn State Hershey Medical Center, 500 University Drive H-091, Hershey, PA 17033, USA
* Corresponding author.
E-mail address: jlighthall@pennstatehealth.psu.edu

Facial Plast Surg Clin N Am 30 (2022) 277–290
https://doi.org/10.1016/j.fsc.2022.03.002

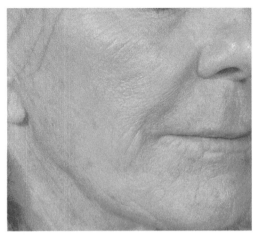

Fig. 1. Photoaged skin. Note the textural irregularities, dyspigmentation, static rhytids, and loss of tone with sagging.

exercise, pollution, and weather issues including wind and temperature extremes. As melanin is protective of ultraviolet exposure, people with darker skin types therefore exhibit fewer signs of photoaging.[4] Extrinsic skin changes include deleterious changes in skin pigmentation, texture, and skin moisture content. These combined changes in the skin begin to manifest as aged inelastic skin secondary to changes in elastin, glycosaminoglycans, and collagen integrity.[7]

The Facial Muscles

Involutional changes in muscle occur throughout the body and manifest themselves as a progressive loss of tone and muscle mass.[8] In the face, secondary to repetitive contraction of the aging muscle in an environment of diminished skin elasticity, soft tissue support mechanisms, and tissue volume loss, one observes hyperdynamic and dysfunctional muscle activity. Over time this creates changes in the soft tissues in different regions of the face. In the upper face, one sees the development of lines that progress from dynamic rhytids to deep permanent furrows. In the central and lower face, these dynamics create the

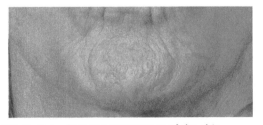

Fig. 2. Peau d'orange appearance of the chin.

downturned oral commissures with marionette lines and the deepening furrows at the nasolabial folds. The contraction of the orbicularis oris muscle that creates the sensuous puckered lips in the youthful face overwhelms the perioral skin and, along with volume loss, creates static radial perioral rhytids and a more tense and pursed appearance in the aged face. Mentalis hypercontraction can lead to the peau d'orange appearance in the chin (Fig. 2).[7,9]

The Facial Soft Tissue Volume

The shape of the face is determined by the underlying skeletal structures and the facial subcutaneous volume. This facial subcutaneous volume to a small degree is composed of the facial muscles but includes to a larger extent the contribution of the facial subcutaneous fat in addition to the deeper fat compartments.[10,11] The superficial musculoaponeurotic system (SMAS) overlies and at some locations intertwines with the mimetic facial muscles and is contiguous with the platysma in the neck. The facial fat is generally regarded as lying in two different planes as superficial and deep in reference to this plane.[12] Both of these layers are further subdivided into smaller fat compartments. The deep fat compartments are closely associated with the underlying bone, are relatively immobile, have different types of adipocytes, and have been speculated to provide a gliding plane for muscle movement (Fig. 3A). The superficial fat compartments are felt to be more mobile and subject to gravitational forces (Fig. 3B).[10] These forces and changes in the facial retaining ligaments that undergo involution or attenuation due to other skeletal volume loss cause soft tissue descent.[13,14] Although ligamentous attachments do not resorb, due to changes in surrounding soft tissue and bony volume and alterations in subcutaneous fat compartments, ligamentous attachments will contribute to the appearance of furrows and grooves throughout the face such as the tear trough deformities, labiomental creases, nasolabial folds, etc (Fig. 4).[12] Facial volume replacement during facial rejuvenation is generally directed to the superficial layer although deeper injections are also used.[15,16]

The Facial Bones

With aging, individuals demonstrate a progressive skeletal regression and remodeling in many regions of the facial skeleton (Fig. 5).[17,18] In the upper face, the forehead flattens along with a decreasing bony volume of the orbital rim thus lowering the eyebrow position and increasing the size of the bony orbit. In the midface, there is a

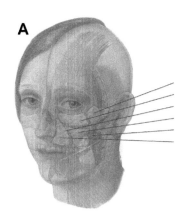

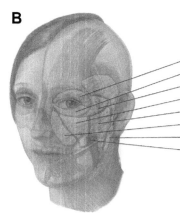

Fig. 3. (*A*) Deep and (*B*) superficial fat compartments of the face. (*From* Gierloff M, Stöhring C, Buder T, Gassling V, Açil Y, Wiltfang J. Aging changes of the midfacial fat compartments: a computed tomographic study. Plastic and reconstructive surgery 2012; 129:263-273.)

A

Sub–orbicularis oculi fat (lateral part)
Sub–orbicularis oculi fat (medial part)
Deep medial cheek fat (medial part)
Deep medial cheek fat (lateral part)
Buccal extension of the buccal fat
Ristow´s space

B

Superior orbital fat
Inferior orbital fat
Lateral orbital fat
Medial cheek fat
Middle cheek fat
Nasolabial fat
Lateral temporal-cheek fat
Buccal extension of the buccal fat

continual and age-related maxillary retrusion and dentoalveolar regression resulting in a flattening of the midface that contributes to the descent of the midfacial soft tissues. The mandible undergoes atrophy in several key areas including a loss of chin projection and wasting along the mandibular ramus, contributing to the loss of lower facial definition, soft tissue ptosis, and prominent grooves. As the facial skeleton is the scaffold for the facial soft tissues, consideration for treatment of the skeleton should be given during facial rejuvenation.[19,20]

Regional Changes in the Aging Face

The upper third of the face

In the upper third of the face, one observes a deepening of the superior orbital sulcus as the size and shape of the orbit expand.[21] There is a wasting and deprojection of the bony orbital rim. The eyebrow descends because of the loss of elasticity and lengthening of the forehead skin and a deflating of the periorbital fat along with the loss of the temporal fat pad. There is a secondary increase of dynamic forehead wrinkles and furrows as the frontalis muscle continuously

contracts to keep the brow elevated allowing a stabilization of vision and the amount of light entering the eyes. Chronic contraction of the procerus and corrugators produce inferior descent of the medial brow and creation of static furrows and dynamic lines. Laterally, the brow becomes ptotic due to the repetitive action of the orbicularis. Laxity and skin excess occur in the eyelids and along with pseudoherniation of orbital fat pads, loss of elasticity, fatiguing of retaining ligaments, and volumetric changes including an expanding bony vault, results in the overall aged appearance of the upper face and periocular region (Fig. 6).[19,22,23]

The middle third of the face

The principal change that is observed in the aging midface is the apparent descent of the cheek soft tissues with loosening of retaining structures and ligaments. This results in a number of undesirable features including skeletonization of the inferior orbital rim and zygoma, pseudoherniation of fat in the lower eyelid, the appearance of the "tear trough" deformity, an apparent deepening of the nasolabial sulcus, laxity of the skin, orbicularis

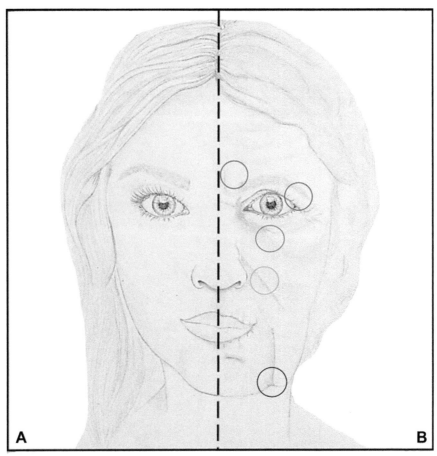

Fig. 4. A youthful (*A*) versus an aged (*B*) face. Circles represent some key areas of aging due to combined repetitive muscle action, skin changes, skeletal and soft tissue volume loss or descent, and positioning of the retaining ligaments. (*From* Cotofana S, Fratila AA, Schenck TL, Redka-Swoboda W, Zilinsky I, Pavicic T. The Anatomy of the Aging Face: A Review. Facial Plast Surg 2016; 32:253-260.)

hypertrophy, and a flattened central upper midface (see **Fig. 6**). The skin of the eyelids thins and loses its elasticity (dermatochalasis) and takes on a crepe-paper appearance with visible subdermal vessels and pigmentary changes. These changes are secondary to the regional skeletal changes, attenuation of the facial retaining ligaments, and actual fat atrophy.[15,16,24]

The lower central third of the face

The central lower face undergoes visible aging changes different than the rest of the face. This is secondary to the prominent changes in the bone and subcutaneous volume loss. There is resorption of bone at the mentum thus reducing mandibular projection. Additional mandibular atrophy is irregularly distributed along various locations of the mandibular margin depending on the underlying biomechanical forces. This is especially pronounced in the area of the anterior mandible immediately inferior to the mental foramina,

resulting in an anatomic bony depression known as the anterior mandibular groove, just anterior to the attachments of the mandibular ligament.[9] With atrophy of the overlying fat compartments and the hypertrophy of the regional musculature one notes characteristic changes in the lower central face including the deepening of the melomental folds, the mental crease, and the labiomandibular creases. The resultant distortions result in anatomic characteristics that we identify as of jowling, the appearance of marionette lines, and a deepening pre-jowl sulcus (**Fig. 7**).

With bony and soft tissue volume loss and repetitive perioral muscular contraction, the lips take on an elongated appearance with static and dynamic rhytids, loss of definition, a flattened or deflated appearance with a poor dental show and oral commissure descent (see **Fig. 1**). In the chin, there is bone loss and soft tissue ptosis with progressive worsening of the skin contour with dimpling causing a peau d'orange

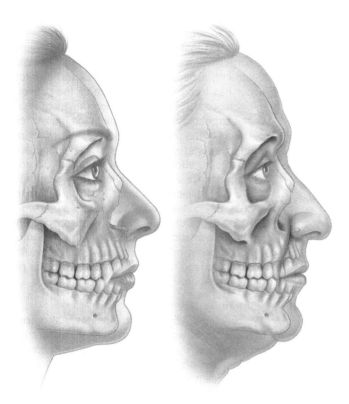

Fig. 5. Skeletal changes that occur with age. (*From* Mendelson B, Wong CH. Changes in the Facial Skeleton With Aging: Implications and Clinical Applications in Facial Rejuvenation. Aesthetic plastic surgery 2020; 44:1151-1158.)

appearance with progression to the "witch's chin" from further severe loss and descent of chin volume and support.

The neck

Underlying anatomy plays a critical role in the aged appearance of the neck as it sets the skeletal framework. Chin and hyoid position will alter the cervicomental angle. Ptosis of the submandibular glands will lead to fullness and less definition below the body of the mandible. Soft tissue ptosis in the lower face and neck along with atrophy of the mandible and fat deposition in the submental region creates a loss of the distinct borders between the lower face and neck with a poorly defined mandibular line (see **Fig. 7**). This is further exacerbated by the appearance of platysmal banding and medial hypertrophy along with excess sagging skin with static horizontal furrows. Loss of skin elasticity and photoaging will affect the overall appearance of face/neck transition and may require treatment to optimize rejuvenation.[25]

PATIENT EVALUATION

In the approach to the patient seeking facial rejuvenation, it is optimal that the practitioner has at their disposal a constellation of noninvasive,

minimally invasive, and more invasive rejuvenation techniques and technologies that they are facile with. Decision-making and recommendations can then be best based on the patient's anatomic and psychological needs rather than on a limited repertoire of technical assets. Together, the history and exam will help the practitioner create a framework for individualized multimodal treatment planning of facial aging.

PATIENT SELECTION AND CANDIDACY FOR FACIAL REJUVENATION

The Motivations of the Patient Seeking Facial Rejuvenation

Psychological motivations

As in all aspects of cosmetic surgery, the surgeon should aim to have a firm understanding of each patient's motivations for undergoing a cosmetic intervention. It is important that these motivations be sound and healthy. One has to be particularly concerned about the patient who is undergoing the intervention as a reaction to or to please another person. For instance, if someone is in the current throes of a divorce, they may not be in the best psychological condition and undergo a procedure that is permanent and has at least a small chance of having a less than optimal recovery.

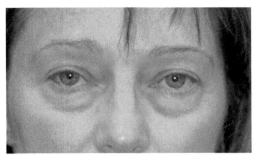

Fig. 6. Aged appearance of eyes with flattened, asymmetric brows, dermatochalasis, blepharoptosis, pseudoherniation of fat, and deep infraorbital hollows.

Social motivations

We are including this heading here because of the current trends of creating "selfies" and the "posting" of such images on social media. One should be careful to properly counsel the patient who has decided to undergo a surgical procedure because how they look in their selfies. On the most elemental level, the patient should be educated that many of the images seen a social media are distorted by various photo and computer factors and do not represent how they actually look.[26] Also emerging is the phenomenon of "zoom dysmorphia" as there has been an increased use of digital platforms with real-time camera use.[27] The outward facial expression may be distorted by computer or smart device angles, lighting, and distance and accentuate true or perceived flaws in the facial form.

Expectations of the patient

What is equally important is to be aware of the patient's understanding of the limitations of various

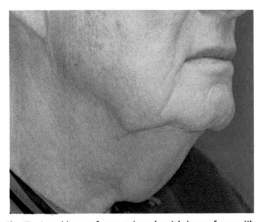

Fig. 7. Aged lower face and neck with loss of mandibular bone and definition, deep marionette lines, downturned oral commissures, prejowl sulcus, moderate jowling, loss of definition of lips, and skin and fat excess in the neck with platysmal banding.

minimally invasive procedures and to establish realistic expectations. If the patient expresses an expectation that they will obtain results similar to a surgical procedure from a minimally invasive treatment, a pause may be in order. The practitioner has to be wary and redirects the patient's expectations. It is extremely important that the patient's expectations are set within the realistic capabilities of the procedure. Screening for patients with unrealistic expectations or a dysfunctional body image, such as body dysmorphic disorder (BDD), which is a preoccupation on physical flaws that are not visible or minimally visible to others, should be considered. Studies have shown a BDD incidence of around 13% in patients presenting with cosmetic concerns. Despite some interventions being minimally invasive, they have the potential to lead to unhappy outcomes in this patient population.[28]

Contraindications

Typical surgical contraindications may also apply to minimally invasive facial rejuvenation. Contraindications such as poor health, inflammatory or autoimmune disease, tobacco abuse, the use of anticoagulants, pregnancy, active illness, and others issues should be considered.

MULTIFACETED AND REGIONAL APPROACH TO FACIAL AGING

A discussion of the multifactorial nature of facial aging is critical for patients to understand the need for a multifaceted approach to optimal rejuvenation addressing their individual aging concerns.[29]

In some situations, the result of a minimally invasive procedure can be quite impressive. For example, the "perfect" lips produced with the use of a hyaluronic acid filler in the younger patient or the elimination of dynamic glabellar wrinkling with a neuromodulator. In many situations, however, the optimal treatment of a facial region will be to use several minimally invasive techniques to produce a balanced or harmonious result (see **Table 1** for a list of common minimally invasive treatments targeting the aging face and neck).

The Rejuvenation of Aged Facial Skin

The treatment of aged skin is aimed at improving texture, pigmentation, and elasticity. There have been many advancements over the last 30 years to rejuvenate the skin.

Medical grade skincare

The most basic fundamental maintenance and rejuvenation regimen directed at the facial skin

Table 1
Common minimally invasive treatments for rejuvenation of the face and neck

Modality	Examples	Desired Effect
Topicals	Retinoids Sunscreens Lightning agents Vitamin/Antioxidants Combination/Compound Therapy	Treatment of lines, texture, elasticity, tone. Increase collagen. Prevention of photoaging Depigmentation Decrease sallowing, improve photoaging and dyschromia Offers multimodal therapy for aging
Treatment of pigment and vascularity	Broadband light Intense pulsed light Pulsed dye laser ND:YAG	Improve hyperpigmentation, fine lines Treat hypervascularity
Chemodenervation	Botox, Dysport, Xeomin, Jeuveau	Smooth dynamic line Lip flip Chemical brow lift
Fillers	Hyaluronic acid Calcium hydroxylapatite Polylactic acid Polymethyl-methacrylate microspheres Platelet-rich plasma Allograft adipose matrix	Restore youthful volume Create symmetry Add lift Static rhytids/grooves Stimulate collagen, elastin, and extracellular matrix
Resurfacing	Ablative vs nonablative vs fractional lasers Dermabrasion Peels	Treatment of lines, texture, elasticity, tone Stimulate collagen synthesis Improve dyspigmentation
Lipolysis	Phosphatidylcholine Deoxycholic acid-injection Transcutaneous cryolipolysis Ultrasound, radiofrequency, or laser-assisted liposuction/lipolysis	Adipose reduction (liposculpture)
Vascular lasers/light therapies	Intense pulsed light Pulsed dye laser Broadband light Nd:YAG	Decrease pigmentation Decrease erythema and prominent vessels
Nonsurgical skin tightening	Ultrasound technology Radiofrequency (monopolar, bipolar, unipolar)	Skin tightening Reduction of wrinkles Fat reduction
Muscle development	Electromagnetic stimulation and direct current	Improve muscle tone
Biostimulants	Biostimulants (eg, growth factor injections, exosomes, platelet-rich plasma poly-L-lactic acid, or calcium hydroxylapatite microspheres)	Increase collagen, elastic and extracellular matrix Reverse photoaging Stimulate volume
Percutaneous collagen induction therapy	Microneedling alone or with biostimulants or radiofrequency	Enhance collagen synthesis and reorientation Dermal thickening
Suture suspension	Thread lifting (polydiaxanone, polyglcolic acid, poly-lactic-polycaprolactone acid, polyproplylene)	Tissue resuspension and tightening Collagen production

should include at least a combination of tretinoin, antioxidants, and sunscreens. Tretinoin will reverse some of the skin photodamage.[30] It will increase the rate of epidermal cell turnover that will restore a more orderly cellular progression from the basal to the keratin layer. This results in an improvement in skin texture and pigmentation. The skin will appear smother and reflect light more efficiently producing a subtle luminescence to the skin. Tretinoin will stimulate collagen synthesis and over time will result in a more orderly array of collagen bundles in the skin.[31] This will result in flattening and improvement in fine rhytids. Elastin synthesis is also increased resulting in a more resilient skin.

The second fundamental is the use of skin antioxidants, such as Vitamin C and E-containing products. They will serve to eliminate free radicals in the skin. Free radicals serve as an intermediary in the process of sunlight-related skin damage. Antioxidants have shown benefits in treating photoaged skin and improving dyschromia.[32]

Although many treatments for photoaging exist, the ideal situation would be to prevent photoaging with avoidance and the appropriate use of sunscreen to reduce the deleterious extrinsic effects of UV radiation on the skin. Additionally, studies have shown that consistent sunscreen use may reverse some of the signs of photoaging.[33]

Other topicals, such as moisturizers or products containing hyaluronic acid and ceramides, may be beneficial for overall skin health.

RESURFACING OF THE SKIN

Skin resurfacing is typically directed at improving wrinkles, texture, and brown pigmentation issues by stimulating a secondary tissue healing response to injury-inducing epithelialization, collagen remodeling, and creation of new collagen and elastin.[6] In the spectrum of resurfacing, there are agents that produce minimal epidermal exfoliation to those that produce near-total ablation of epidermis and partial removal of the dermis. Resurfacing may be performed with chemical agents (peels), mechanical agents (dermabrasion and microdermabrasion), and a variety of energy and light-based therapies such as lasers and plasma devices. For brevity, we will largely refrain from a thorough discussion of the spectrum of agents available and instead touch on laser and energy devices.

The earlier full ablative CO_2 and erbium lasers created tighter and smoother skin but could hardly be considered minimally invasive and could easily result in a patient "healing' time of several weeks with increased risk of texture irregularities, fine

scarring, and pigment concerns. Fractional laser technologies made it possible to create skin that was improved and retained a normal texture, pigmentation and architecture. Newer advances in laser technology using picosecond technologies and different wavelengths have produced results with limited rates of complications, impressive skin tightening and a better targeting of pigmentation and vascular defects with a limited downtime of hours to days (**Fig. 8**).[34,35]

Treatment of Skin Vascular and Pigmented Lesions

Although the ablation of the skin epithelium will many times improve hyperpigmented lesions of the facial skin, the treatment of vascular lesions and benign pigmented lesions of the skin are many times addressed differently than the management of rhytids in the skin. The 595 nm pulsed dye laser and the 1064 nm long-pulsed Nd:YAG has been used for the management of a variety of vascular lesions such as port-wine stains and telangiectasias. Hyperpigmented lesions are frequently managed with erbium and picosecond Nd:YAG lasers (see **Fig. 8**). Intense pulse light and other lasers are is also used (see **Table 1**).[36]

The Rejuvenation of Facial Volume and Contour

Skin tightening—energy devices

Skin tightening devices have become popular. Underlying technologies include ultrasound, helium plasma, and radiofrequency stimulation of the skin. The core mechanism of skin tightening in all of these devices is the heating of the dermis and subdermal structures to induce a secondary healing response. A reactionary collagen synthesis is induced with resultant contraction and skin tightening. This is done in a manner without ablation of the skin or a prolonged downtime. Skin tightening then occurs over weeks to months.

Percutaneous and transcutaneous devices are available. Some of these devices provide tightening as well as subcutaneous fat remodeling. Serial treatments are typically required to obtain improvement. Commonly used devices to achieve these goals incorporate ultrasound technology, plasma, and monopolar, bipolar, or unipolar radiofrequency (**Fig. 9**).[37–39] More recently, several noninvasive energy devices have been introduced to induce skin tightening of the face and neck without any penetration of the skin or subcutaneous tissues (**Fig. 10**). Preliminary reports and experience are optimistic. The long-term effects and longevity of these treatments are still unknown (**Figs. 11 and 12**).

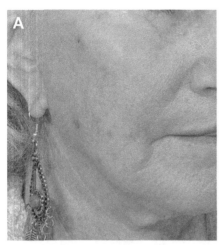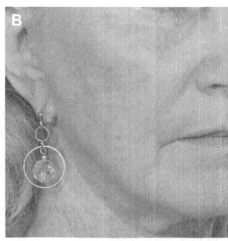

Fig. 8. Clinical images depicting improvement of facial lentigines and modest skin tightening with single treatment picosecond 1064/532 nm laser (PicoLazer, Rohrer Aesthetics). Treatment resulted in approximately 24 hours of "redness" downtime. (*A*) Pretreatment, (*B*) Post-Treatment.

Suture suspension

Although treatments are available for skin tightening, resurfacing, fat reduction, or volume rejuvenation, ptotic soft tissue may still be a problem.[40] To combat this, soft tissue suture suspension was developed as a minimally invasive technique. Multiple types of suture are now available, with both nonabsorbable and absorbable threads on the market. The ideal patient is younger without advanced signs of aging. For optimal rejuvenation, thread lifting may be combined with other minimally invasive therapies.[41]

Treatment of dynamic rhytids

The neuromodulators occupy a unique position in the esthetic ecosystem of facial rejuvenation. Their sole mechanism of action is to weaken or *modulate* muscle contraction. When used in strategic areas, with many areas being off-label, the neuromodulators can be used esthetically to lessen glabellar frown lines, decrease forehead motion, soften periorbital rhytids, passively elevate the brows, and improve the oral commissure position. Their high efficiency and low complication rate make the neuromodulators extremely popular and safe to use.

Restoring facial volume and treatment of static lines/furrows

Among the most significant changes in the aging face is the loss and malposition of facial volume. Although replacement of volume with alloplastic implants or autologous fat transfer is still commonly performed, the most significant change has been through the introduction of injectable fillers. The use of off-the-shelf fillers and biostimulatory agents is now among the most commonly performed esthetic procedures.

The injectable filler availability has grown immensely since the introduction of Restylane in 2003 as the first hyaluronic acid filler.[42] The hyaluronic acid fillers currently garner the largest proportion of the market and use as they have an excellent safety profile, are easy to use, and are reversible. As a sole treatment, filler is ideal in younger patients or to treat deep grooves (**Fig. 13**) or enhance lips. Autogenous fat transfer has become more popular, may be performed under local, and may be combined with tightening procedures (see **Fig. 11**).[24,43–46]

Biostimulants, stem cells, and exosomes

In recent decades, an interest has developed in biostimulants and stem cells for the induction of collagen and elastin production and extracellular matrix to combat photoaging (see **Table 1**).[47,48] These may be used as adjuncts with other minimally invasive therapies or as volume replacement.

Lipolysis

Some areas retain fat that is resistant to weight loss and may show increased deposition with age. To combat this, multiple nonsurgical techniques have been developed, including deoxycholic acid injection, transcutaneous cryolipolysis, and ultrasound-assisted lipolysis.[49]

TREATMENT PLANNING

Treatment planning should be an interactive process between patient and practitioner. Patients now present having done more "research" that

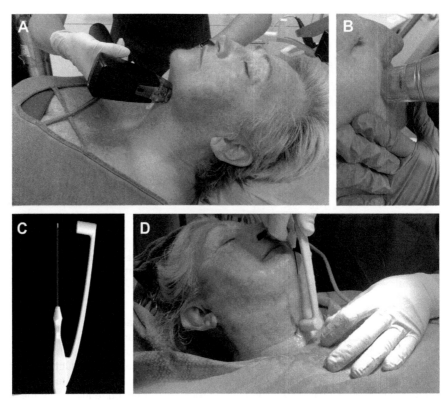

Fig. 9. Transcutaneous radiofrequency microneedling devices. (*A*) Morpheous 8 (Inmode, Inc.), (*B*) Pixel8 (Rohrer Aesthetics), (*C*) percutaneous radiofrequency device (FaceTite handpiece, Inmode, Inc.), and (*D*) clinical image of FaceTite being used for local lipolysis and skin tightening of neck.

may not be correct or ideal for their situation. It is therefore paramount that the clinician attempts to guide the patient to develop an individualized treatment plan.

In the passages that follow, we will briefly discuss the regional rejuvenation of one's face from the perspective that we are specifically *not* going to recommend surgery but instead use the spectrum of interventions in the minimally invasive range. Keep in mind that there are many variations on this theme and what is offered here is a series of

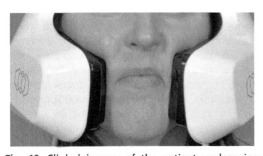

Fig. 10. Clinical images of the patient undergoing noninvasive lower facial skin tightening with one of the two Evoke devices (Inmode, Inc.).

interventions that has worked in our practices. As it is in many cases, even when the full spectrum of interventions is being entertained, it is helpful to ascertain the face in terms of regions and address what might be done from region to region. These treatments will be discussed in more detail in other articles on this issue.

A FACIAL REGIONAL APPROACH TO THE USE OF NONINVASIVE AND MINIMALLY INVASIVE THERAPIES
The Upper Face

Patients frequently seek consultation for rejuvenation of the upper face related to aging issues such as forehead wrinkles, brow ptosis, dermatochalasis, glabella furrows, and periorbital rhytids. Other issues that can be identified at the time of consultation include temporal fat wasting, hollowing of the superior orbital sulcus, skeletonization of the superior orbital rims, skin laxity, lentigines, rhytids, and poor texture.[22]

Among the most popular and effective vehicles for rejuvenation of the upper face are neuromodulators for dynamic lines. Although Botox (Allergan Aesthetics) still commands a market dominance,

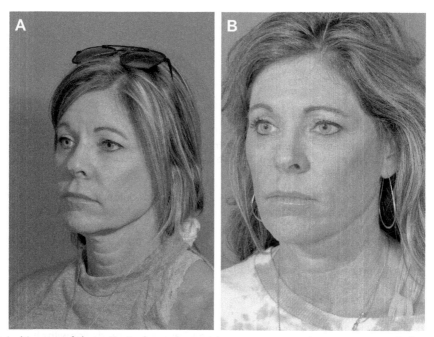

Fig. 11. Clinical images of the patient who underwent transcutaneous and percutaneous radiofrequency treatment of face and neck and fat transfer. (A) Preoperative and (B) postoperative.

other alternatives are available and are arguably just as effective. In the upper facial region, the selective weakening of the brow depressors will facilitate frontalis muscle elevation actions thus

resulting in an elevation of the eyebrows and providing a chemical brow lift. Treating the forehead, periocular region, and glabella can diminish dynamic forehead wrinkles and furrows. Patient

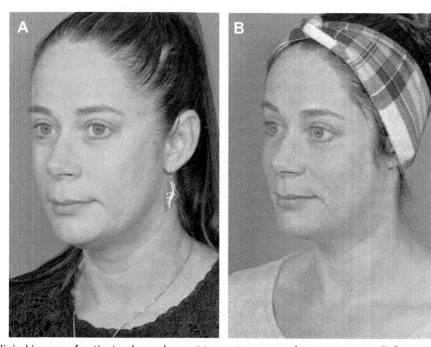

Fig. 12. Clinical images of patients who underwent transcutaneous and percutaneous radiofrequency treatment of lower eyelid fat pseudoherniation and simultaneous with single treatment picosecond 1064/532 nm laser treatment of regional face and neck skin. (A) Preprocedure and (B) postprocedure.

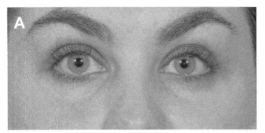
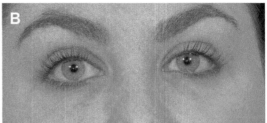

Fig. 13. Clinical images of patients who underwent correction of tear trough deformity with the injection of a total of 1 cc of Kysse (Galderma, Inc.). (*A*) Preprocedure and (*B*) postprocedure.

selection and strategic use of the neuromodulators are important in this location as if overdone they can cause a secondary brow or lid ptosis.

Fillers, autogenous fat, and biostimulants may be used to minimize the appearance of deep furrows in the glabella, forehead, and periorbital region and can be used to add volume to skeletonized brows and orbital rims and minimize temporal hollowing.

Photoaged skin may be treated with any of the resurfacing techniques, prominent vessels may be minimized with the use of vascular-directed lasers, and tightening may be obtained by ultrasound or radiofrequency techniques (see **Figs. 11** and **12**).

The Midface

The descent of the midface soft tissues results in the skeletonization of the infraorbital rim and development of a tear trough deformity, deepening of the nasolabial groove, and flattening of the upper midface. The ptosis of the upper central midface results in the biconvexity deformity (see **Fig. 6**).

The use of injectable volume agents including fillers, biostimulating products, and fat transfer all have excellent track records for the rejuvenation of the midface. Adding volume to the deep at the malar eminence and upper midface, filling in the nasojugal groove and tear-trough, and softening of the nasolabial fold (see **Fig. 13**).

Minimally invasive skin tightening, suture suspension, and treatment of photoaged skin may be treated with a combination of skincare products, thread lifting, radiofrequency, microneedling, resurfacing, and use of vascular lasers (see **Figs. 11** and **12**).

The Lower Face and Lips

Although neuromodulation at the upper vermilion border or in the depressor anguli oris muscles may be beneficial to improve radial perioral lines, provide a "lip flip" or turn up low oral commissures, this is not the primary modality in this region. Instead, a combination of fillers to minimize the appearance of grooves and contour the chin and mandibular, resurfacing to treat textural irregularities and induce collage production, and tightening devices to provide definition are the mainstay (see **Fig. 11**).

Neck

Minimally invasive treatments to rejuvenate the neck are aimed at minimizing excess fat with liposculpting, treating surface irregularities with resurfacing, minimizing dynamic rhytids with chemodenervation, and tightening of skin and soft tissue. The lower face and mandible are typically treated in conjunction to re-establish the mandibular line and provide a more youthful, defined transition.

SUMMARY

Although minimally invasive techniques have revolutionized facial rejuvenation when used or alone or, more commonly, in combination, there are limitations to what can be achieved through these techniques and patients must be counseled about realistic expectations. The vast majority of these modalities available are valid and effective. The clinician's job is to choose among this constellation of interventions that best suit the patient's individual desires and needs anatomically and psychologically.

CLINICS CARE POINTS

- A multimodal approach to facial aging will provide optimal rejuvenation results.
- Treatments plans should be individualized based on patient goals and aging characteristics and may include skin care regimens, minimally invasive therapies, and surgical interventions.
- Proper patient evaluation and counseling are critical components of a holistic approach to facial rejuvenation.

REFERENCES

1. American Society of Plastic Surgeons: Plastic Surgery Statistics Report 2020. Available at: https://www.plasticsurgery.org/documents/News/Statistics/2020/plastic-surgery-statistics-full-report-2020.pdf.
2. Gerth DJ. Structural and volumetric changes in the aging face. Facial Plast Surg 2015;31:3–9.
3. Flament F, Bazin R, Laquieze S, et al. Effect of the sun on visible clinical signs of aging in Caucasian skin. Clin Cosmet Investig Dermatol 2013;6:221–32.
4. Vashi NA, de Castro Maymone MB, Kundu RV. Aging Differences in Ethnic Skin. J Clin Aesthet Dermatol 2016;9:31–8.
5. Fedok FG. The aging face. Facial Plast Surg 1996;12:107–15.
6. Fisher GJ, Varani J, Voorhees JJ. Looking older: fibroblast collapse and therapeutic implications. Arch Dermatol 2008;144:666–72.
7. Swift A, Liew S, Weinkle S, et al. The Facial Aging Process From the "Inside Out. Aesthet Surg J 2021;41:1107–19.
8. Campbell MJ, McComas AJ, Petito F. Physiological changes in ageing muscles. J Neurol Neurosurg Psychiatry 1973;36:174–82.
9. Fedok FG, Mittelman H. Augmenting the Prejowl: Deciding between Fat, Fillers, and Implants. Facial Plast Surg 2016;32:513–9.
10. Gierloff M, Stöhring C, Buder T, et al. Aging changes of the midfacial fat compartments: a computed tomographic study. Plast Reconstr Surg 2012;129:263–73.
11. Rohrich RJ, Pessa JE. The fat compartments of the face: anatomy and clinical implications for cosmetic surgery. Plast Reconstr Surg 2007;119:2219–27.
12. Cotofana S, Fratila AA, Schenck TL, et al. The Anatomy of the Aging Face: A Review. Facial Plast Surg 2016;32:253–60.
13. Furnas DW. The retaining ligaments of the cheek. Plast Reconstr Surg 1989;83:11–6.
14. Brandt MG, Hassa A, Roth K, et al. Biomechanical properties of the facial retaining ligaments. Arch Facial Plast Surg 2012;14:289–94.
15. Yang CS, Huang YL, Chen CB, et al. Aging Process of Lateral Facial Fat Compartments: A Retrospective Study. Aesthet Surg J 2021;41:NP247–54.
16. Gosain AK, Klein MH, Sudhakar PV, et al. A volumetric analysis of soft-tissue changes in the aging midface using high-resolution MRI: implications for facial rejuvenation. Plast Reconstr Surg 2005;115:1143–52 [discussion: 1153–5].
17. Mendelson B, Wong CH. Changes in the Facial Skeleton With Aging: Implications and Clinical Applications in Facial Rejuvenation. Aesthet Plast Surg 2020;44:1151–8.
18. Richard MJ, Morris C, Deen BF, et al. Analysis of the anatomic changes of the aging facial skeleton using computer-assisted tomography. Ophthalmic Plast Reconstr Surg 2009;25:382–6.
19. Kahn DM, Shaw RB Jr. Aging of the bony orbit: a three-dimensional computed tomographic study. Aesthet Surg J 2008;28:258–64.
20. Shaw RB Jr, Kahn DM. Aging of the midface bony elements: a three-dimensional computed tomographic study. Plast Reconstr Surg 2007;119:675–81 [discussion: 682–3].
21. Neimkin MG, Holds JB. Evaluation of Eyelid Function and Aesthetics. Facial Plast Surg Clin North Am 2016;24:97–106.
22. Fedok FG. The Aesthetics of the Upper Face: Forehead, Brow, and Upper Eyelid. Facial Plast Surg 2018;34:107–8.
23. Truswell WHt. Aging changes of the periorbita, cheeks, and midface. Facial Plast Surg 2013;29:3–12.
24. Tzikas TL. Autologous fat grafting for midface rejuvenation. Facial Plast Surg Clin North Am 2006;14:229–40.
25. Koch RJHM. Aesthetic Facial Analysis. In: Papel EbID, editor. Facial plastic and reconstructive surgery. 3rd edition. New York: Thieme; 2008. p. 177–87.
26. Chen J, Ishii LE, Liao D, et al. Selfies and Surgery: How Photo Editing Impacts Perceptions of Facial Plastic Surgery Capabilities. Facial Plast Surg Aesthet Med 2021;23:393–4.
27. Gasteratos K, Spyropoulou GA, Suess L. Zoom Dysmorphia": A New Diagnosis in the COVID-19 Pandemic Era? Plast Reconstr Surg 2021;148:1073e–4e.
28. Wever CCC, Wever A, Constantian M. Psychiatric Disorders in Facial Plastic Surgery. Facial Plast Surg Clin North Am 2020;28:451–60.
29. Fedok FG. Facial Rejuvenation: A Multidimensional and Multimodal Perspective. Facial Plast Surg 2021;37:139.
30. Hubbard BA, Unger JG, Rohrich RJ. Reversal of skin aging with topical retinoids. Plast Reconstr Surg 2014;133:481e–90e.
31. Griffiths CE, Russman AN, Majmudar G, et al. Restoration of collagen formation in photodamaged human skin by tretinoin (retinoic acid). N Engl J Med 1993;329:530–5.
32. Fitzpatrick RE, Rostan EF. Double-blind, half-face study comparing topical vitamin C and vehicle for rejuvenation of photodamage. Dermatol Surg 2002;28:231–6.
33. Randhawa M, Wang S, Leyden JJ, et al. Daily Use of a Facial Broad Spectrum Sunscreen Over One-Year Significantly Improves Clinical Evaluation of Photoaging. Dermatol Surg 2016;42:1354–61.

34. Cortez EA, Fedok FG, Mangat DS. Chemical peels: panel discussion. Facial Plast Surg Clin North Am 2014;22:1–23.

35. Fedok FG, Garritano F, Portela A. Cutaneous lasers. Facial Plast Surg Clin North Am 2013;21:95–110.

36. Heidari Beigvand H, Razzaghi M, Rostami-Nejad M, et al. Assessment of Laser Effects on Skin Rejuvenation. J Lasers Med Sci 2020;11:212–9.

37. Han X, Yang M, Yin B, et al. The Efficacy and Safety of Subcutaneous Radiofrequency After Liposuction: A New Application for Face and Neck Skin Tightening. Aesthet Surg J 2021;41:NP94–100.

38. Gold MH, Biron J. Improvement of wrinkles and skin tightening using TriPollar((R)) radiofrequency with Dynamic Muscle Activation (DMA). J Cosmet Dermatol 2020;19:2282–7.

39. Kaplan H, Kaplan L. Combination of microneedle radiofrequency (RF), fractional RF skin resurfacing and multi-source non-ablative skin tightening for minimal-downtime, full-face skin rejuvenation. J Cosmet Laser Ther 2016;18:438–41.

40. Moon H, Fundaro SP, Goh CL, et al. A review on the combined use of soft tissue filler, suspension threads, and botulinum toxin for facial rejuvenation. J Cutan Aesthet Surg 2021;14:147–55.

41. Fundaro SP, Goh CL, Hau KC, et al. Expert consensus on soft-tissue repositioning using absorbable barbed suspension double-needle threads in asian and caucasian patients. J Cutan Aesthet Surg 2021;14:1–13.

42. Restylane FDA approval letter. Available at: https://www.accessdata.fda.gov/cdrh_docs/pdf4/p040024a.pdf.

43. Fedok FG. The Rejuvenation of the Aged Central Lower Face: A Contemporary Perspective. Facial Plast Surg 2019;35:121–8.

44. Chang CS, Kang GC. Achieving ideal lower face aesthetic contours: combination of tridimensional fat grafting to the chin with masseter botulinum toxin injection. Aesthet Surg J 2016;36(10):1093–100.

45. Braz A, Humphrey S, Weinkle S, et al. Lower Face: Clinical Anatomy and Regional Approaches with Injectable Fillers. Plast Reconstr Surg 2015;136:235S–57S.

46. Metzinger S, Parrish J, Guerra A, et al. Autologous fat grafting to the lower one-third of the face. Facial Plast Surg 2012;28:21–33.

47. Miller-Kobisher B, Suárez-Vega DV, Velazco de Maldonado GJ. Epidermal growth factor in aesthetics and regenerative medicine: systematic review. J Cutan Aesthet Surg 2021;14:137–46.

48. Peng GL. Platelet-rich plasma for skin rejuvenation: facts, fiction, and pearls for practice. Facial Plast Surg Clin North Am 2019;27:405–11.

49. Talathi A, Talathi P. Fat Busters: Lipolysis for Face and Neck. J Cutan Aesthet Surg 2018;11:67–72.

Photoaging and Topical Rejuvenation

Katherine Berry, MD, Katherine Hallock, MD, Charlene Lam, MD, MPH*

KEYWORDS

• Photoaging • Skin rejuvenation • Sunscreen • Tretinoin • Hydroquinone • Alpha hydroxy acid
• Topical niacinamide • Topical vitamin C

KEY POINTS

• Photoaging is a complex process of skin changes including rhytids, lentigines, telangiectasias, mottled pigmentation, coarse texture, and laxity caused by chronic ultraviolet exposure.
• Strict photoprotection with sunscreen is the best defense for photoaging.
• Topical retinoids are the cornerstone for an antiaging topical regimen.
• Combination topicals should be used with caution as the stability and absorption are questionable when compounded.
• Hydroquinone, the most commonly used and studied lightning agent, should be used with physician oversight due to possible adverse effects.

INTRODUCTION

The skin is the most visible indicator of aging. Ultraviolet (UV) light, specifically UVA, and the cumulative exposure are the main culprits of photoaging. Clinically, photoaging can be appreciated as rhytids, telangiectasias, dyspigmentation, volume loss, and even malignancy.[1] On a microscopic level, there is a reduction in epidermal thickness, pigment heterogeneity, dermal elastosis, collagen degradation, ectatic vessels, and mutagenesis of keratinocytes and melanocytes.[1] The purpose of topicals is to help reduce and reverse these signs of aging and restore the organ to its highest functioning level. Although easily overlooked, a topical regimen is the foundation for facial rejuvenation. The number of topicals and the claims of efficacy can be overwhelming especially with the number of over-the-counter cosmeceuticals. It is impractical for a physician to be familiar with all available products on the market so focus will be placed on a core group of medical grade, evidence-based topicals including retinoids, lightning agents, and other vitamin/antioxidant agents. We will discuss our approach for optimal skin care regimens and routines.

SUNSCREEN

Up to 80% of aging can be attributed to UV exposure.[2] Thus, limiting sun exposure and protecting the skin from UV radiation is paramount for the prevention of facial aging and maintenance of rejuvenation measures. Solar UV radiation consists of UVA (320–400 nm), UVB (280–320 nm), and UVC (100–280 nm). UVC fails to reach the Earth's surface as it is completely absorbed by the ozone layer.[3] Historically, UVB was thought to be the major contributor to photoaging. It is predominantly absorbed by the epidermis, and it composes the major portion of UV radiation that induces sunburns and erythema.[3] However, UVA, which is 20 times more abundant than UVB at the level of the Earth's surface,[4] has a longer wavelength. This leads to deeper dermal penetration and has been found to be the primary driver of photoaging.[5] For example, when there is chronic, asymmetric exposure of the face to UVA radiation, the exposed side has a clinically increased level of skin wrinkling and roughness .[6] Additionally, in

Department of Dermatology, Penn State Health Hershey Medical Center, Hershey, PA, USA
* Corresponding author. Department of Dermatology, Penn State Health, 500 University Drive, HU14, Hershey, PA 17033.
E-mail address: clam@pennstatehealth.psu.edu

Facial Plast Surg Clin N Am 30 (2022) 291–300
https://doi.org/10.1016/j.fsc.2022.03.003

skin of color patients, UVA radiation leads to irregular skin pigmentation, which is associated with photoaging in this population.[5] Currently there is mounting evidence that both visible and infrared light also play a role in photoaging and pigmentary changes. The visible light spectrum extends from 400 to 700 nm and has been found to stimulate matrix metalloproteinase production, which leads to the degradation of dermal collagen.[7] Furthermore, studies suggest a synergistic effect between UVA radiation and visible light in driving age-related pigmentary changes.[8,9]

Although the skincare market often focuses on products that reverse skin aging, it is much more efficacious to focus on prevention .[10] Sun avoidance and sun-protective clothing, such as hats and shirts may be helpful, in limiting UV damage, but sunscreens remain the mainstay of facial photoprotection. Sunscreens have historically been split into two major categories, physical (inorganic) and chemical (organic) blocking agents. Both types of agents work via absorption of UV radiation. Spectrums of absorption vary in chemical agents and typically a combination of organic filters is necessary in order to provide protection across the full range of UV radiation. As visible light is now implicated in photoaging and dyspigmentation, there is an increased interest in protection against these wavelengths. However, this can be difficult to achieve with cosmetically acceptable results, as these sunscreens must be opaque in order to block visible light.[11,12] Notably, only pigmentary grade zinc oxide and titanium dioxide protect against visible light and not the micronized forms.[12] Iron oxide and pigmentary titanium dioxide are the most commonly used visible light filters, and they are used in tinted formulations that may be matched to an individual's skin tone.[11,12]

Sun protection factor (SPF), is the standard for measuring the protective ability of a sunscreen. This is based on UV-induced erythema, which, is mostly UVB driven. In order to account for UVA radiation, sunscreens can be labeled as broad spectrum if greater than 90% of UVA is absorbed at $\geq$ 370 nm.[13] There are currently no guidelines for visible light protection, and as iron oxide is not an Food and Drug Administration (FDA) approved inorganic filter, it is listed as an inactive ingredient on sunscreen labels.

There is high-quality evidence that daily sunscreen prevents of photoaging.[14,15] A study including 903 adults randomized to daily sunscreen application versus discretionary sunscreen application tracked participants over 4.5 years. At the end of the study period, the daily sunscreen group showed no detectable increase in skin aging, which was 24% less than skin aging in the discretionary sunscreen group.[14] Daily sunscreen application has been suggested to reverse signs of extrinsic aging.[16] A study of 32 patients who applied daily broad-spectrum SPF 30 sunscreen over a 1 year period showed significantly improved skin clarity, pigmentation, and texture in all subjects.[16] Studies examining the benefit of visible light protection have been primarily performed in the setting of melasma.[17,18] In a double-blind study of 68 female subjects with melasma, there was a significant improvement in Melasma Area Severity Index (MASI) and Physician's Global Assessment scores in those who applied UV and visible light filters, including iron oxides, versus UV filters alone.[18]

Although there has been recent controversy over the safety of sunscreens due to systemic absorption,[19,20] a systematic review in 2020 showed no evidence of human health risk,[21] and its benefits are thought to outweigh the theoretic risks. There has also been concern over the environmental impact on coral reefs, but most studies have shown sunscreen concentrations are lower than the required threshold for coral reef toxicity.[22] However, there have been a few studies that demonstrated oxybenzone and octinoxate, which are both organic sunscreens, have some risk on coral reef health.[23] Sunscreens with these filters are banned in certain locations. This is an area that requires further research. It is important to note that physical blockers, such as zinc oxide and titanium dioxide, have not demonstrated health or environmental risk, and they have achieved Category I- generally recognized as safe and effective (GRASE) by the FDA.[24]

It is generally recommended that a tinted, broad spectrum, SPF 30+ sunscreen be used on a daily basis to provide protection against UV radiation and visible light in order to reduce the effects of photoaging.[25] Even if one is mostly indoors, sunscreen application is still critical, as UVA radiation penetrates through glass,[4] and visible and blue light are ubiquitous in our environment. Additionally, sunscreen should be reapplied every 2 hours, as well as after sweating or water exposure.

RETINOIDS

Topical retinoids, used as monotherapy and in combination, are the cornerstone of treatment for photoaging. Its efficacy and use in photoaging have been well reviewed.[26–28] As a class of compounds related to vitamin A (eg, retinol, retinyl esters, retinaldehyde), it is converted to its most biologically active form, trans-retinoic acid. The mechanism of action involves diffusion into the cell and transportation into the nucleus by the cellular retinol-binding proteins or cellular retinoic acid-binding proteins. Within the nucleus, the retinoid binds to the retinoic acid receptor or to the retinoid X receptor, which act as ligand-dependent transcription factor. This allows either increases or decreases in the expression of specific proteins and enzymes.[28]

Historically, tretinoin was used to treat several dermatologic conditions, most commonly acne, and it was observed to have an effect on photoaging.[29] Evidence demonstrating the effectiveness of topical retinoids for aging has been shown clinically, histologically, and at the molecular level.[28] Clinically, it reduces the appearance of fine/coarse lines, improves skin texture, improves tone and elasticity, and slows photoaging.[26,30] Histologically, it has been shown to increase collagen production,[31] induce epidermal hyperplasia, and decrease keratinocyte and melanocytic atypia.[32] Molecularly, it increases collagen syntheses via inhibition of UV-induced c-Jun and alternation of TGF-beta expression, inhibition of collagen degradation via matrix metalloproteinases (MMP) inhibition, increased epidermal proliferation and differentiation, inhibits tyrosinase activity, and increases glycosaminoglycans (GAG), which binds water, increasing epidermal hydration.[33]

Of the topical compounds, tretinoin is the most widely used and studied compound. As the beneficial effects of tretinoin on photodamaged skin cease after discontinuation , it is recommended that initial topical treatment is maintained by long-term use. The most studied concentration of tretinoin is 0.05%. In one study, tazarotene compared with tretinoin 0.05% provided a more rapid response; however, at the conclusion the study period there was no difference in overall improvement.[34] Topical over- the- counter retinols have been shown to improve photodamage such as epidermal thickening and increase collaged synthesis.[35] However, its potency is 20-fold less compared with retinoic acid. Although retinols can be less irritating than retinoic acid, it is also very unstable, degrading into inactive metabolites.[36] That is important to keep in mind when recommending over-the-counter products.

Many patients often abandon the use of topical retinoids before reaping the beneficial effects. A minimum of 3 months use is required to appreciate epidermal changes. Dermal changes are not seen until 9–12 months. Therefore, it is important to prescribe the correct formulation, coach patients through the side effects, and manage their expectations (Table 1). Retinoid dermatitis and photosensitivity can be seen in the beginning of treatment. Common side effects include erythema, burning, stinging, dryness, and scaling.

To improve tolerability, initiate retinoid at the lowest strength of 0.025%. Encourage moisturizer use at least 30 minutes after retinoid application and start with thrice-weekly application and increase to daily as tolerated. There also are novel vehicle delivery systems that improve tolerability such as liposomes, controlled-delivery systems, and nanoparticles.[26]

HYDROQUINONE

Hydroquinone is the gold standard of depigmenting agents and is effective in the treatment of melasma and hyperpigmentation. Hydroquinone acts by binding histidines on the active site of tyrosinase.[37] Tyrosinase is the rate-limiting step in melanin production by melanocytes. Furthermore, hydroquinone reduces DNA and RNA synthesis by glutathione depletion, resulting in melanosome degradation.[38] It has also been shown to selectively damage melanosomes and melanocytes.[39]

Hydroquinone comes in a variety of concentrations, but the 4% strength is most commonly used in dermatology practices. A randomized, placebo-controlled trial of 48 patients showed significant improvement in pigmentation in hydroquinone 4% treated patients compared with placebo.[40] Additionally, 40% of hydroquinone patients had complete resolution of their hyperpigmentation. Klingman first proposed that hydroquinone's skin lightning effects may be further enhanced by the addition of corticosteroids and retinoids.[41] His original formulation was hydroquinone 5%, tretinoin 0.1%, and dexamethasone 0.1%, and this combination of active ingredients has been continually replicated. Corticosteroids decrease irritation caused by hydroquinone and tretinoin and tretinoin stimulates cell turnover and hydroquinone penetration.[42] A multicenter, randomized controlled trial of 260 subjects over 8 weeks showed that a triple combination cream of fluocinolone acetonide 0.01%, hydroquinone 4%, and tretinoin 0.05% had superior efficacy in comparison to hydroquinone 4% alone in the treatment of melasma.[43] However, the triple therapy group did have a higher rate of skin irritation. In addition, a 2010 Cochrane systematic review including 2125 participants showed that triple combination cream was more effective at lightning melasma than hydroquinone cream alone.[44] Although more high-quality studies are needed to further determine the ideal formulation and parameters for clinical use.

In addition to skin irritation, the most common side effect, there are several more concerning adverse effects. Although uncommon, exogenous ochronosis, the permanent deposition of yellow-

Table 1
Side effects of topical retinoids and ways to increase tolerance

Side Effect	Advice
Dryness	• Emollient moisturizer 30 min AFTER application of retinoid • Emollient moisturizer with SPF in the morning
Irritation	• Wait 30 min after washing face • Apply every other night to build up tolerance eventually increasing to every night • Apply after the face is completely dry • Avoid chemical or physical scrubs • Pea-size amount to the whole face
Redness	• Strict sun protection
Stinging	• Avoid chemical or physical scrubs • Liposome or nanoparticle carrier
Sensitive skin (eg, Fitzpatrick type 1, historical intolerance to perfumes, chemical sunscreens, or astringents, atopic dermatitis, rosacea)	• Initiate tretinoin at0.025% qHS

pigmented fibers within the dermis is a feared complication. This clinically appears as reticulated blue-grey macules in treated areas. It can be almost prevented with the appropriate use of hydroquinone.[45] A systematic review showed that the development of exogenous ochronosis occurred after a median duration of use of 5 years, and only four cases were reported when using hydroquinone for 3 months or less.[45] Additionally, exogenous ochronosis was more frequently reported when hydroquinone concentrations were greater than 4%. Additional risk factors include Black race and Fitzpatrick skin types V and VI, both being associated with greater than 50% of exogenous ochronosis cases. Although extremely rare, there is a risk of permanent depigmentation due to oxidative damage to membrane lipids in melanocytes.[46] Only eight cases have been reported in the literature of hydroquinone causing permanent leukoderma.[47] There have been significant safety concerns with hydroquinone due to it being a benzene derivative and reports of animals developing malignancy after being treated for extended periods with high oral doses.[48] It is currently banned in Europe, Australia, and Japan although there have been no reports of cutaneous or internal malignancy associated with hydroquinone in humans over its 40 to 50 years of clinical use.[49]

Up until 2020, hydroquinone was available over the counter in a 2% formulation. As part of the Coronavirus Aid, Relief, and Economic Security Act, hydroquinone was categorized as not non-GRASE, eliminating over-the-counter sales. It remains available as a prescription product and is commonly compounded into a triple therapy

cream. Of note, there is only one FDA-approved product containing hydroquinone (Tri-Luma, Galderma Labs), which also contains tretinoin and fluocinolone. When compounding hydroquinone, it can be difficult to formulate in a stable preparation as it rapidly oxidizes. Hydroquinone will change from a creamy color to dark yellow or brown as oxidation occurs, making it less efficacious. Therefore, any products with color change should be replaced.[50]

We feel that hydroquinone applied topically as a thin layer one to two times daily for up to 3 months has a good safety profile. Being mindful to avoid overtreatment and ensuring drug holidays may be helpful in preventing side effects. Additionally, concomitant use of sun protective measures to prevent further hyperpigmentation is critical.

NIACINAMIDE

Niacinamide is an active form of vitamin B3 that has become increasingly popular in skincare products. Its physiologic role is as a precursor to nicotinamide adenine dinucleotide and its phosphate derivative (NADPH). These cofactors and their reduced forms (NADH and NADPH) function as coenzymes in many redox reactions. The reduced forms also act as antioxidants in the skin. It has been shown that topical niacinamide readily penetrates human skin and increases local levels of NADH after topical application.[51] It has also been shown to increase collagen and GAG production, which can help to decrease wrinkling by boosting these dermal matrix components. Additionally, niacinamide increases ceramide levels of the skin, as NADPH is a cofactor in the synthesis of fatty acids and lipids, which in turn enhances the skin's barrier function.[52]

Clinical studies have supported the effectiveness of niacinamide on improving visible signs of aging.[53,54] In a randomized, double-blind, placebo-controlled trial of 50 white females with clinically apparent photodamage, niacinamide 5% was applied twice daily for 12 weeks to half of the face, although a vehicle control was applied to the other half. The niacinamide-treated skin showed significantly reduced redness, lightning of hyperpigmentation, and decreased sallowness.[55] Sallowness, or age-related yellowing of the skin, is due to the Maillard reaction. This reaction involves spontaneous oxidation and glycation of proteins, the rate of which increases with age. The resulting cross-linked proteins lead to a yellow tint to the skin. Niacinamide is specifically beneficial in the reduction of sallowing, as its antioxidant forms, NADH and NADPH, inhibit the Maillard reaction, and thus, reduce skin sallowing.[54] This has been supported clinically by several studies that showed a significant reduction in sallowness after the application of topical niacinamide.[53,55]

Daily to twice daily application of niacinamide-containing products is typically well tolerated. Concentration varies based on formulation, and there is evidence that the antiaging effects of niacinamide are dose dependent, as improvement with niacinamide 5% was significantly better than 2%.[56] Although topical niacinamide has not shown the same efficacy in photoaging improvement as retinoids, it lacks skin irritation and is thus suitable for patients with sensitive skin.[53] It can also be used in addition to a regimen with other potentially irritating products. Furthermore, it has not been shown to have any inflammatory or carcinogenic properties.[57]

VITAMIN C

Vitamin C is a popular cosmeceutical ingredient and is the most plentiful and important antioxidant in the skin.[58] Vitamin C plays an essential role in transcription and post-translation collagen synthesis and has been shown to downregulate MMP responsible for collagen degradation.[59] Vitamin C also reduces inflammation and UV-induced immunosuppression.[58] Moreover, vitamin C inhibits melanogenesis and resulting hyperpigmentation by inhibiting copper ions on tyrosinase active sites.[59]

Several studies have shown that topical application of vitamin C improves the appearance of photoaging and dyspigmentation[59–63]; however, oral supplementation remains controversial.[64] In one double-blind, placebo-controlled trial, subjects who applied 10% topical vitamin C over 12 weeks had a statistically significant reduction in photoaged scores and skin wrinkling.[62] Skin biopsies also revealed increased grenz zone type 1 collagen. Another double-blind, placebo-controlled trial involving 6 months of vitamin C 5% application looking at structural improvements revealed improved skin furrowing on histology, along with improved clinical appearance.[61]

Most studies evaluating topical vitamin C benefits in dyspigmentation have evaluated its use in melasma. An open-label study evaluating 40 melasma patients applying L-ascorbic acid 25% for 16 weeks revealed a significant decrease in MASI scores, improvement in skin pigmentation as evaluated by mexameter and improvement in melasma specific quality of life index.[65] When compared to hydroquinone 4%, ascorbic acid 5% had similar improvements in colorimetry; however, more patients in the hydroquinone group had good and excellent results based on photography and patient report.[66]

Vitamin C most commonly occurs in its active form, L-ascorbic acid, which is unstable and hydrophilic. Therefore, L-ascorbic acid has poor skin penetration due to the hydrophobic nature of the stratum corneum.[67] Reducing the pH of L-ascorbic acid by the addition of ferulic acid improves stability and permeability due to transformation into a hydrophobic molecule.[67,68] Additional studies have looked at the use of vitamin C esters, which are active and have an added benefit of being nonirritating.[69] Regardless of formulation, vitamin C must be in its active form and should have a concentration of 8% to 20% in order to have a biologically significant effect.[67] In concentrations greater than 20%, there is no improved d cutaneous absorption and higher concentrations are associated with increased irritation.[67]

ALPHA HYDROXY ACID

The use of alpha-hydroxy acids is a centuries-old practice to improve skin appearance, dating back to ancient Egyptian medicine and initially described in the Ebers Papyrus in 1550 BC..[70] Queen Cleopatra was famously known to bathe in sour milk to improve the texture and cosmesis of her skin.[71] Unbeknownst to her, the active ingredient was lactic acid, an alpha-hydroxy acid. Alpha hydroxy acids include glycolic acid, lactic acid, malic acid, citric acid, pyruvic acid, tartaric acid, and other less commonly known acids. They are hydrophilic organic acids with a carboxylic acid moiety and an adjacent hydroxyl acid group in the alpha position. Although the exact mechanism of action remains unknown, they are

Table 2
Additional products for specific complaints

Patient Concern	Addition to Topical Routine
Dull/sallowness	• Vitamin C q am before sunscreen
Sensitive skin	• Niacinamide q am • Sunscreen with physical blockers only
Pigment (melasma; lentigines; postinflammatory hyperpigmentation)	• Hydroquinone q pm (can be compounded with tretinoin)
Coarse/roughness	• Alpha hydroxy acid

[a]Core topical regimen involves sunscreen in the morning and retinoid in the evening.

thought to function via epidermolysis. By removing calcium ions from epidermal cell adhesions via chelation, they result in the weakening of adhesions resulting in an exfoliative effect.[72] Additionally, they have been shown to increase collagen and hyaluronic acid within the dermis.[73]

Although most studies involving the use of alpha hydroxy acids have been performed with chemical peeling, evaluation of their use in leave-on products has also been performed in small studies. Ditre and colleagues recruited 17 volunteers in a split arm study with moderate to severe photoaging.[74] They applied a 25% glycolic acid, lactic acid, or citric acid lotion to one forearm versus vehicle on the other arm. After 6 months, they found the alpha hydroxy acid group had increased skin thickness, reversal of basal cell atypia, melanin dispersal, normal rete, increased papillary dermal thickness with increased collagen density, and improved elastic fiber quality. Further studies have also reported improvement in wrinkling, roughness, and dyspigmentation with the daily application of leave-on alpha hydroxy acids.[75–77]

The daily application of alpha hydroxy acid-containing compounds in concentrations up to 20% appears to be well tolerated.[78] Adverse effects depend on the concentration and pH of the product used. Potential mild negative side effects include skin irritation, stinging, burning, pain, and erythema. Side effects become more frequent and severe with increasing concentration; therefore concentrations up to 70% and a pH 2 or less should be restricted to professional use.[78]

OUR APPROACH

Topicals have a role in priming the skin before other surgical rejuvenation procedures.[27] It has been shown that pretreatment with retinoid creams before chemical peels and dermabrasion improved the uniformity of frosting and reepithelialization. However, short-term pretreatment before carbon dioxide laser has not demonstrated benefit in reepithelialization or hyperpigmentation.

Moreover, although some providers recommend hydroquinone pretreatment before rejuvenation procedures in those with an increased risk of postinflammatory hyperpigmentation, there is insufficient data to demonstrate that pretreatment hydroquinone can diminish this risk.

The essential components of a topical skincare routine are sun protection and a retinoid. Although seemingly straightforward, achieving routine use of these products is easier prescribed than done by patients. Furthermore, the number of over-the- counter cosmeceuticals is overwhelming and challenging to assess efficacy. As they are not classified as drugs, they are not subject to the rigorous testing and regulation of the FDA. Many of the combination creams are proprietary so it can be difficult to compare products. As indicated above, many of the components discussed can become unstable and inactivate easily. Although the over- the- counter anti-aging creams can serve as moisturizers, we tend to recommend bland, emollient moisturizers to combat the irritation of the prescription strength retinoids. Combined sunscreens and moisturizers are convenient to use in the mornings and establish a routine. As for retinoids, our recommendation is to familiarize oneself with a few retinoids for the different skin types and common complaints that prevent adherence. Other agents can be added for specific concerns (**Table 2**). In our experience, a simple routine increases compliance and tolerability, which is key as these topicals are intended for lifelong maintenance and prevention.

SUMMARY

The skin is the most visible indicator of aging. The major extrinsic factor that causes aging is UV light. Optimizing skin health with a topical routine with photoprotection and retinoid is the foundation of facial rejuvenation. Due to the irritability of prescription strength retinoids and length of time needed for results, adherence is an issue even though their efficacy has been demonstrated on the clinical, histologic, and molecular levels. Coaching patients through the side effects and choosing a well-tolerated retinoid is key. Furthermore, without strict photoprotection, any topical will be counterproductive.

CLINICS CARE POINTS

- Regardless of the skin type or pigmentation, daily photoprotection best prevents the aging effects of UVA.
- Long-term use of topical retinoids can reduce the appearance of fine/coarse lines, improves skin texture, improves tone and elasticity, and slows photoaging.
- Hydroquinone inhibits melanin production and can treat hyperpigmentation. Caution must be used when determining the concentration and length of time used.
- Niacinamide, an active form of vitamin B3, can lessen redness, hyperpigmentation, and sallowness, reducing signs of photoaging. Although not a potent as retinoids, it is less irritating.
- Topical application of vitamin C improves the appearance of photoaging and dyspigmentation. The active form is unstable and has poor penetration of the stratum corneum.
- Alpha hydroxyl acids have an exfoliative effect and can reduce coarseness.
- Keep topical routines simple to reduce irritation and augment compliance.

DISCLOSURE

K. Berry and K. Hallock have no disclosures. C. Lam serves on the Clinical Council for Genentech, Inc.

REFERENCES

1. Yaar M, Gilchrest BA. Photoageing: mechanism, prevention and therapy. Br J Dermatol 2007; 157(5):874–87.
2. Flament F, Bazin R, Laquieze S, et al. Effect of the sun on visible clinical signs of aging in Caucasian skin. Clin Cosmet Investig Dermatol 2013;6:221.
3. Young AR, Claveau J, Rossi AB. Ultraviolet radiation and the skin: Photobiology and sunscreen photoprotection. J Am Acad Dermatol 2017;76(3):S100–9.
4. Wang F, Smith NR, Tran BAP, et al. Dermal Damage Promoted by Repeated Low-Level UV-A1 Exposure Despite Tanning Response in Human Skin. JAMA Dermatol 2014;150(4):401–6.
5. Battie C, Jitsukawa S, Bernerd F, et al. New insights in photoaging, UVA induced damage and skin types. Exp Dermatol 2014;23:7–12.
6. Mac-Mary S, Sainthillier JM, Jeudy A, et al. Assessment of cumulative exposure to UVA through the study of asymmetrical facial skin aging. Clin Interv Aging 2010;5:277. Accessed October 18, 2021./ pmc/articles/PMC2946854/.
7. Cho S, Lee MJ, Kim MS, et al. Infrared plus visible light and heat from natural sunlight participate in the expression of MMPs and type I procollagen as well as infiltration of inflammatory cell in human skin in vivo. J Dermatol Sci 2008;50(2):123–33.
8. Kohli I, Chaowattanapanit S, Mohammad TF, et al. Synergistic effects of long-wavelength ultraviolet A1 and visible light on pigmentation and erythema. Br J Dermatol 2018;178(5):1173–80.
9. Ruvolo E, Fair M, Hutson A, et al. Photoprotection against visible light-induced pigmentation. Int J Cosmet Sci 2018;40(6):589–95.
10. Poon F, Kang S, Chien AL. Mechanisms and treatments of photoaging. Photodermatol Photoimmunology Photomed 2015;31(2):65–74.
11. Geisler AN, Austin E, Nguyen J, et al. Visible light. Part II: Photoprotection against visible and ultraviolet light. J Am Acad Dermatol 2021;84(5):1233–44.
12. Lyons AB, Trullas C, Kohli I, et al. Photoprotection beyond ultraviolet radiation: A review of tinted sunscreens. J Am Acad Dermatol 2021;84(5):1393–7.
13. Wang SQ, Xu H, Stanfield JW, et al. Comparison of ultraviolet A light protection standards in the United States and European Union through in vitro measurements of commercially available sunscreens. J Am Acad Dermatol 2017;77(1):42–7.
14. Hughes MCB, Williams GM, Baker P, et al. Sunscreen and prevention of skin aging: A randomized trial. Ann Intern Med 2013;158(11):781–90.
15. Boyd AS, Naylor M, Cameron GS, et al. The effects of chronic sunscreen use on the histologic changes of dermatoheliosis. J Am Acad Dermatol 1995;33(6):941–6.
16. Randhawa M, Wang S, Leyden JJ, et al. Daily Use of a Facial Broad Spectrum Sunscreen over One-Year Significantly Improves Clinical Evaluation of Photoaging. Dermatol Surg 2016;42(12):1354–61.
17. Boukari F, Jourdan E, Fontas E, et al. Prevention of melasma relapses with sunscreen combining protection against UV and short wavelengths of visible light: A prospective randomized comparative trial. J Am Acad Dermatol 2015;72(1):189–90.e1.
18. Castanedo-Cazares JP, Hernandez-Blanco D, Carlos-Ortega B, et al. Near-visible light and UV photoprotection in the treatment of melasma: a double-blind

randomized trial. Photodermatol Photoimmunology Photomed 2014;30(1):35–42.

19. Matta MK, Zusterzeel R, Pilli NR, et al. Effect of Sunscreen Application Under Maximal Use Conditions on Plasma Concentration of Sunscreen Active Ingredients: A Randomized Clinical Trial. JAMA 2019;321(21):2082–91.

20. Matta MK, Florian J, Zusterzeel R, et al. Effect of Sunscreen Application on Plasma Concentration of Sunscreen Active Ingredients: A Randomized Clinical Trial. JAMA 2020;323(3):256–67.

21. Suh S, Pham C, Smith J, et al. 13382 Two banned sunscreen ingredients and their impact on human health: A systematic review. J Am Acad Dermatol 2020;83(6):AB7.

22. Mitchelmore CL, Burns EE, Conway A, et al. A Critical Review of Organic Ultraviolet Filter Exposure, Hazard, and Risk to Corals. Environ Toxicol Chem 2021;40(4):967–88.

23. Abbasi J. FDA Trials Find Sunscreen Ingredients in Blood, but Risk Is Uncertain. JAMA 2020;323(15):1431–2.

24. Federal Register :: Sunscreen Drug Products for Over-the-Counter Human Use. Available at: https://www.federalregister.gov/documents/2019/02/26/2019-03019/sunscreen-drug-products-for-over-the-counter-human-use. Accessed October 26, 2021.

25. Guan LL, Lim HW, Mohammad TF. Sunscreens and Photoaging: A Review of Current Literature. Am J Clin Dermatol 2021;1–10. https://doi.org/10.1007/S40257-021-00632-5.

26. Mukherjee S, Date A, Patravale V, et al. Retinoids in the treatment of skin aging: an overview of clinical efficacy and safety. Clin Interv Aging 2006;1(4):327–48.

27. Hubbard BA, Unger JG, Rohrich RJ. Reversal of skin aging with topical retinoids. Plast Reconstr Surg 2014;133(4). https://doi.org/10.1097/PRS.0000000000000043.

28. Darlenski R, Surber C, Fluhr JW. Topical retinoids in the management of photodamaged skin: from theory to evidence-based practical approach. Br J Dermatol 2010;163(6):1157–65.

29. Kligman AM, Grove GL, Hirose R, et al. Topical tretinoin for photoaged skin. J Am Acad Dermatol 1986;15(4 Pt 2):836–59.

30. Cho S, Lowe L, Hamilton TA, et al. Long-term treatment of photoaged human skin with topical retinoic acid improves epidermal cell atypia and thickens the collagen band in papillary dermis. J Am Acad Dermatol 2005;53(5):769–74.

31. Griffiths C, Russman AN, Majmudar G, et al. Restoration of collagen formation in photodamaged human skin by tretinoin (retinoic acid). New Engl J Med 1993;329(8):530–5.

32. Bhawan J, Olsen E, Lufrano L, et al. Histologic evaluation of the long term effects of tretinoin on photodamaged skin. J Dermatol Sci 1996;11(3):177–82.

33. Fisher GJ, Voorhees JJ. Molecular mechanisms of retinoid actions in skin. Fed Am Societies Exp Biol J 1996;10(9):1002–13.

34. Kang S, Krueger GG, Tanghetti EA, et al. A multicenter, randomized, double-blind trial of tazarotene 0.1% cream in the treatment of photodamage. J Am Acad Dermatol 2005;52(2):268–74.

35. Varani J, Warner RL, Gharaee-Kermani M, et al. Vitamin A antagonizes decreased cell growth and elevated collagen-degrading matrix metalloproteinases and stimulates collagen accumulation in naturally aged human skin. J Invest Dermatol 2000;114(3):480–6.

36. Kang S, Duell EA, Fisher GJ, et al. Application of retinol to human skin in vivo induces epidermal hyperplasia and cellular retinoid binding proteins characteristic of retinoic acid but without measurable retinoic acid levels or irritation. J Invest Dermatol 1995;105(4):549–56.

37. Palumbo A, d'Ischia M, Misuraca G, et al. Mechanism of inhibition of melanogenesis by hydroquinone. Biochim Biophys Acta 1991;1073(1):85–90.

38. Gillbro JM, Olsson MJ. The melanogenesis and mechanisms of skin-lightning agents – existing and new approaches. Int J Cosmet Sci 2011;33(3):210–21.

39. Jimbow K, Obata H, Pathak MA, et al. Mechanism of Depigmentation by Hydroquinone. J Invest Dermatol 1974;62(4):436–49.

40. Ennes SBP, Paschoalick RC, Alchorne MMDA. A double-blind, comparative, placebo-controlled study of the efficacy and tolerability of 4% hydroquinone as a depigmenting agent in melasma. J Dermatol Treat 2000;11(3):173–9.

41. Kligman AM, Willis I. A new formula for depigmenting human skin. Arch Dermatol 1975;111(1):40–8.

42. Guevara IL, Pandya AG. Melasma treated with hydroquinone, tretinoin, and a fluorinated steroid. Int J Dermatol 2001;40(3):212–5.

43. Chan R, Park KC, Lee MH, et al. A randomized controlled trial of the efficacy and safety of a fixed triple combination (fluocinolone acetonide 0·01%, hydroquinone 4%, tretinoin 0·05%) compared with hydroquinone 4% cream in Asian patients with moderate to severe melasma. Br J Dermatol 2008;159(3):697–703.

44. Rajaratnam R, Halpern J, Salim A, et al. Interventions for melasma. Cochrane Database Syst Rev 2010;7. https://doi.org/10.1002/14651858.CD003583.PUB2.

45. Ishack S, Lipner SR. Exogenous ochronosis associated with hydroquinone: a systematic review. Int J Dermatol 2021. https://doi.org/10.1111/IJD.15878.

46. Arndt KA, Fitzpatrick TB. Topical Use of Hydroquinone as a Depigmenting Agent. JAMA 1965;194(9):965–7.

47. Jow T, Hantash BM. Hydroquinone-induced depigmentation: case report and review of the literature.

Dermatitis 2014;25(1). https://doi.org/10.1097/01. DER.0000438425.56740.8A.

48. Nordlund, JJ. (2007). Hydroquinone: its value and safety. Commentary on the US FDA proposal to remove hydroquinone from the over-the-counter market. Expert Review of Dermatology, 2(3), 283–287.

49. Nordlund J, Grimes P, Ortonne J. The safety of hydroquinone. J Eur Acad Dermatol Venereol 2006; 20(7):781–7.

50. Draelos ZD. Skin lightning preparations and the hydroquinone controversy. Dermatol Ther 2007;20(5): 308–13.

51. Bissett DL. Topical niacinamide provides skin aging appearance benefits while enhancing barrier function. J Clin Dermatol 2003;32:9–18. Available at: https://ci. nii.ac.jp/naid/10023919175. Accessed October 18, 2021.

52. Matts P. A Review of the range of effects of niacinamide in human skin Visual perception and assessment of human skin condition View project Visual perception and assessment of human hair View project. Published online 2002. Available at: https://www.researchgate.net/publication/ 286270242. Accessed October 18, 2021.

53. Bissett DL, Oblong JE, Berge CA. Niacinamide: A B Vitamin that Improves Aging Facial Skin Appearance. Dermatol Surg 2005;31(7 Pt 2):860–6.

54. Wolff S, Jiang Z, Hunt J. Protein glycation and oxidative stress in diabetes mellitus and ageing. Free Radic Biol Med 1991;10(5):339–52.

55. Bissett DL, Miyamoto K, Sun P, et al. Topical niacinamide reduces yellowing, wrinkling, red blotchiness, and hyperpigmented spots in aging facial skin1. Int J Cosmet Sci 2004;26(5):231–8.

56. Matts PJ, Solenick ND. Predicting visual perception of human skin surface texture multiple-angle reflectance. In: Presented at: The 59th Annual Meeting of the American Academy of Dermatology. 2001. Available at: https://www.mendeley.com/guides? dgcid=Mendeley_Desktop_Help-Online-guides. Accessed October 26, 2021.

57. On-Line INFOBASE - ingredients - regulations - labeling ooomctics - personal care products. Available at: https://online.personalcarecouncil.org/jsp/ IngredInfoSearchResultPage.jsp?searchLetter=H& CIRR=WO98JR3. Accessed October 26, 2021.

58. Matsui MS, Hsia A, Miller JD, et al. Non-Sunscreen Photoprotection: Antioxidants Add Value to a Sunscreen. J Invest Dermatol Symp Proc 2009;14(1):56–9.

59. Al-Niaimi F, Chiang NYZ. Topical Vitamin C and the Skin: Mechanisms of Action and Clinical Applications. J Clin Aesthet Dermatol 2017;10(7):14. Accessed October 18, 2021./pmc/articles/PMC56 05218/.

60. Kameyama K, Sakai C, Kondoh S, et al. Inhibitory effect of magnesium l-ascorbyl-2-phosphate (VC-

PMG) on melanogenesis in vitro and in vivo. J Am Acad Dermatol 1996;34(1):29–33.

61. Humbert PG, Haftek M, Creidi P, et al. Topical ascorbic acid on photoaged skin. Clinical, topographical and ultrastructural evaluation: double-blind study vs. placebo. Exp Dermatol 2003;12(3):237–44.

62. Fitzpatrick RE, Rostan EF. Double-Blind, Half-Face Study Comparing Topical Vitamin C and Vehicle for Rejuvenation of Photodamage. Dermatol Surg 2002;28(3):231–6.

63. Traikovich SS. Use of Topical Ascorbic Acid and Its Effects on Photodamaged Skin Topography. Arch Otolaryngol Head Neck Surg 1999;125(10): 1091–8.

64. McArdle F, Rhodes LE, Parslew R, et al. UVR-induced oxidative stress in human skin in vivo: effects of oral vitamin C supplementation. Free Radic Biol Med 2002;33(10):1355–62.

65. Hwang SW, Oh DJ, Lee D, et al. Clinical Efficacy of 25% l-Ascorbic Acid (C'ensil) in the Treatment of Melasma. J Cutan Med Surg 2009;13(2):74–81.

66. Espinal-Perez LE, Moncada B, Castanedo-Cazares JP. A double-blind randomized trial of 5% ascorbic acid vs. 4% hydroquinone in melasma. Int J Dermatol 2004;43(8):604–7.

67. Pinnell SR, Yang H, Omar M, et al. Topical L-Ascorbic Acid: Percutaneous Absorption Studies. Dermatol Surg 2001;27(2):137–42.

68. Lin FH, Lin JY, Gupta RD, et al. Ferulic Acid Stabilizes a Solution of Vitamins C and E and Doubles its Photoprotection of Skin. J Invest Dermatol 2005; 125(4):826–32.

69. Perricone NV. The photoprotective and anti-inflammatory effects of topical ascorbyl palmitate. J Geriatr Dermatol 1993;1(1):5–10. https://doi.org/ 10.2310/7750.2008.07092. https://scholar.google. com/scholar?hl=en&as_sdt=0%2C39&q=PERRI CONE+1993+ascorbyl&btnG=. Accessed October 26, 2021.

70. Smith GE. Ancient Egyptian medicine: the papyrus ebers. Chicago: Ares Publishers; 1930.

71. Rajanala S, Vashi NA. Cleopatra and Sour Milk—The Ancient Practice of Chemical Peeling. JAMA Dermatol 2017;153(10):1006.

72. Wang X. A theory for the mechanism of action of the α-hydroxy acids applied to the skin. Med Hypotheses 1999;53(5):380–2.

73. Bernstein EF, Lee J, Brown DB, et al. Glycolic Acid Treatment Increases Type I Collagen mRNA and Hyaluronic Acid Content of Human Skin. Dermatol Surg 2001;27(5):429–33.

74. Ditre CM, Griffin TD, Murphy GF, et al. Effects of α-hydroxy acids on photoaged skin: Apilot clinical, histologic, and ultrastructural study. J Am Acad Dermatol 1996;34(2):187–95.

75. Stiller MJ, Bartolone J, Stern R, et al. Topical 8% Glycolic Acid and 8% L-Lactic Acid Creams for the

Treatment of Photodamaged Skin: A Double-blind Vehicle-Controlled Clinical Trial. Arch Dermatol 1996;132(6):631–6.

76. Smith WP. Comparative effectiveness of α-hydroxy acids on skin properties. Int J Cosmet Sci 1996; 18(2):75–83.

77. DiNardo JC, Grove GL, Moy LS. Clinical and Histological Effects of Glycolic Acid at Different Concentrations and pH Levels. Dermatol Surg 1996;22(5): 421–4.

78. Babilas P, Knie U, Abels C. Cosmetic and dermatologic use of alpha hydroxy acids. J Dtsch Dermatol Ges 2012;10(7):488–91.

Hyaluronic Acid Basics and Rheology

Grace T. Wu, MD[a], Joanna Kam, MD[b], Jason D. Bloom, MD[a,c],*

KEYWORDS

- Hyaluronic acid • Rheology • Dermal filler

KEY POINTS

- Hyaluronic acid (HA) is the most common dermal filler material used today.
- HA improves wrinkles and volume loss not only by filling and volumizing but also by hydrating the injected area with its water affinity.
- HA is a naturally occurring component of skin, and there is a negligible risk of immunologic or allergic reaction with injection. It is rapidly degraded by the injection of hyaluronidase, thus creating an ideal injectable material that is low risk and reversible.
- Duration of effect may be longer than expected based on bioavailability of the HA product due to collagen synthesis or fibroblast stimulation.

INTRODUCTION

The aging face comprises many commonly observed characteristics including rhytid formation in the glabella and periorbital regions, deepening of the nasolabial grooves, formation of marionette lines, brow ptosis, periorbital and temporal hollowing, atrophy and descent of the midfacial fat pads, and jowling. These changes typically progress in a predictable fashion and are predominantly driven by 3 distinct processes: 1) loss of soft tissue elasticity, 2) gravity-mediated descent of normal structures, and 3) loss of volume.

Loss of volume may be the primary process driving some age-related changes.[1,2] Cadaver studies by Rohrich and colleagues[3] delineate the facial fat compartments, which become more discrete as age-related volume loss occurs. These compartments are both superficial and deep to the facial musculature, and the location predicts how the compartment ages. In general, the superficial fat pads tend to become ptotic or sag, whereas the deep fat pads tend to atrophy or lose volume. Volume loss may occur early in the aging process,[4] and volume restoration with soft tissue fillers can adequately address volume loss without the need for invasive surgical procedures during the early stages of aging.[1,2,5,6]

Injectable soft tissue fillers are widely used to address areas of facial volume loss and wrinkles. Many materials are available on the market, including hyaluronic acid (HA), calcium hydroxylapatite, poly-L-lactic acid, and polymethyl methacrylate. Autologous fat is also commonly used, often in conjunction with surgical procedures. In 2020, the United States (US) HA-based dermal fillers market was estimated at $1 billion and is projected to grow.[7] With numerous products available on the market, and increasing interest in facial rejuvenation, in-depth knowledge of fillers will be critical to providing optimal treatment. This article will discuss HA dermal fillers, the most popular type of dermal filler, and their rheologic characteristics.

BACKGROUND

HA is found in all human tissues, but most abundantly in the skin, synovial fluid, vitreous of the eye, and umbilical cord. The monomeric unit that

[a] Department of Otorhinolaryngology, University of Pennsylvania, 3737 Market Street, Suite 302, Philadelphia, PA 19104, USA; [b] Georgia Center for Facial Plastic Surgery, 613 Ponder Place Drive, Evans, GA 30809, USA; [c] Bloom Facial Plastic Surgery, Two Town Place, Suite 110, Bryn Mawr, PA 19010, USA
* Corresponding author.
E-mail address: DrJBloom@bloomfps.com

Facial Plast Surg Clin N Am 30 (2022) 301–308
https://doi.org/10.1016/j.fsc.2022.03.004

composes HA chains is identical regardless of origin–animal or bacterial–and therefore, there is a negligible risk of immunologic or allergic reaction with HA injection.[8] About half of the total body's HA resides in the skin.[9]

Before the development of HA fillers, collagen was the preferred dermal filler for decades, having obtained Food and Drug Administration (FDA) approval in 1981. However, the collagen was usually derived from a bovine source, and before receiving this treatment, patients required 2 rounds of skin allergy testing.[10] This delay and the potential adverse side effects contributed to why HA dermal fillers rapidly became more popular. Restylane® (Galderma Laboratories) was the first HA filler to be approved by the FDA in 2003 and was initially marketed to address deep wrinkles and folds and later for lip enhancement.[11,12] Of note, HA dermal fillers had been used in Europe for several years before US FDA approval. Shortly after Restylane's FDA approval, many other products came onto the US market, with various characteristics and indications. These products are associated with a low risk of allergic reaction and do not require skin testing before injection.[13]

The filling effect of HA is not only due to direct addition of gel volume to the dermis or subdermis. Studies were conducted based on observations that HA fillers create results lasting beyond what was expected. Its water affinity and the ability to bind large amounts of water contributes to its volumizing effect. In addition, HA dermal fillers have been shown to result in increased collagen stimulation and deposition and increased fibroblast activity around the injected filler.[14,15] Therefore, the duration of effect may be longer than expected based on how long it takes to degrade in vivo.

CHEMICAL COMPOSITION AND MANUFACTURING

HA is a naturally occurring compound in the skin that is an essential component of the extracellular matrix of all adult animal tissues. The HA compound is a glycosaminoglycan disaccharide composed of alternately repeating units of D-glucuronic acid and N-acetyl-D-glucosamine.[15]

In the past, HA was extracted from rooster combs but currently manufacturing of the compound is performed mostly via bacterial fermentation.[16] This process produces uncross-linked HA of varying lengths. The HA chains must next undergo a stabilization process to prevent rapid in vivo enzymatic and oxidative degradation. In order to produce viable dermal HA, nonmodified HA is cross-linked to create a polymer network.[17] 1,4-butanediol diglycidyl ether (BDDE) is the cross-

linker in all of the current FDA-approved HA filler products, including the Restylane® and Juvéderm® (Allergan Aesthetics) families of products, as well as Belotero® Balance (Merz Aesthetics).[18] After the cross-linking step, each manufacturer uses a proprietary technology to modify their products, unique to each line of filler. **Table 1** lists the approximate cross-linking percentage for the FDA-approved HA fillers available at this time.

PHYSICO-CHEMICAL CHARACTERISTICS AND RHEOLOGY
Physico-Chemical Characteristics

The manufacturing process for various commercially available HA fillers has direct implications for the unique gel properties and clinical applications of these products. These gel properties can be described using the science of rheology, which describes the consistency and flow properties of matter, including liquids and soft solids such as gels. Rheologic properties are determined with a rheometer, which consists of 2 nondeformable plates, one fixed and one mobile. A gel is placed between these 2 plates, such that there is complete contact between the gel and the plates. Through manipulation of the mobile plate, properties of the gel can be determined.[5]

There are many physico-chemical characteristics of HA that determine how it behaves. Notably, an injectable product needs to be able to flow through an appropriately sized needle with reasonable extrusion forces. HA is an excellent lubricant in its uncross-linked form, and the presence of uncross-linked HA in a gel facilitates extrusion of the gel through a thin needle into the soft tissues.[17]

The key clinically relevant characteristics to be aware of when selecting a filler are degree of cross-linking, HA concentration, swelling factor, elastic modulus (G′), G″, G*, and tan δ.

Cross-linking
As noted above, cross-linking of HA molecules is an essential step in producing dermal fillers that resist normal enzymatic and oxidative degradation. The degree of cross-linking refers to how many links are between 2 HA molecules on an average. For example, a 4% degree of cross-linking would indicate that there are 4 cross-linker molecules for every 100 disaccharide monomeric units of HA.[17] In the US, BDDE is the only cross-linking agent used. BDDE can react at both ends to link 2 separate strands of HA, resulting in a cross-link. However, the BDDE may bond only at one end, leaving its other end free. This is termed a pendant cross-link.

Table 1
Cross-linking percentage of FDA-approved hyaluronic acid fillers

Product	Percentage Cross-linked
Restylane® Restylane Lyft Restylane Silk	~1.2%
RHA® 2 RHA 3 RHA 4	~3% ~3.5% ~4%
Juvéderm® Ultra Restylane Refyne	~6%
Revanesse® Versa Restylane Kysse Restylane Contour	~7%
Juvéderm Ultra Plus Restylane Defyne	~8%
Juvéderm Voluma Juvéderm Volbella Juvéderm Vollure	Highly cross-linked (proprietary)

Belotero® Balance uses cohesive polydensified matrix technology and percentage cross-linking cannot be measured.

The degree of modification of a gel is determined by the percent of cross-links summed with the percent of pendant modifications. Although cross-linking generally results in firmer and longer-lasting gels, pendant modifications result in softer gels with an increased degree of swelling.[6] Too high a degree of cross-linking or pendant modifications can lead to problems with biocompatibility because the more a given HA product is cross-linked, the more it is altered or modified from HA in its natural form. In products with a significantly higher degree of cross-linking, the body perceives those fillers as more "foreign" and is more likely to cause an immunologic reaction, creating delayed onset swelling and inflammatory nodules. Furthermore, HA fillers with a high degree of cross-linking are longer lasting and may be more difficult to reverse with hyaluronidase because the network is more tightly woven and difficult to access, when exposed to hyaluronidase. When hyaluronidase enzymatically breaks down individual HA molecules in a highly cross-linked gel, the separated pieces may still be attached to the HA polymer network via cross-links, making the overall filler more difficult to break down or dissolve. Pendant modifications do not contribute to longevity.

Hyaluronic acid concentration
HA concentration is defined as the total weight of HA per milliliter (mL) of finished product, typically expressed in milligrams (mg) per mL. See **Table 2** for the reported HA concentrations of FDA-approved fillers. The concentration matters because, in general, the higher it is, the more water a gel needs to incorporate in order to reach equilibrium hydration. The total weight includes both cross-linked and uncross-linked, or free, molecules. Only cross-linked HA resists in vivo degradation and contributes to the longevity of the gel, so it is important to note what percentage of a filler's HA concentration is cross-linked. Free HA is degraded by the body in a matter of days.

Swelling factor
Swelling factor is closely related to HA concentration. HA is hydrophilic and can hold many times its weight in water, leading to increased volume and turgor. One gram of HA can bind up to 6 L of water.[19] It may seem like a higher concentration of HA is desirable; however, if the product is not at or close to equilibrium hydration, it will have a significant amount of tissue water affinity and water uptake once injected. Water may be added to an HA gel, or the HA gel may sit in a dialysis bath, during the manufacturing process to allow it to reach equilibrium hydration. However, it is beneficial for a dermal filler to be slightly below equilibrium hydration because it will then draw in some tissue water and add to the volumizing effect. The swelling factor seems to be linearly related to HA concentration, with the higher concentration HA gels pulling in more tissue water and causing more swelling. Conversely, the swelling factor is inversely related to the degree of cross-linking, as higher degrees of cross-linking reduce the hydrophilicity of a gel. This may limit the volumizing and lifting capacity of the gel.[17]

Rheologic Measurements

Elastic modulus
The elastic or storage modulus is designated G prime (G'). This measurement corresponds to gel firmness and is a measure of a product's ability to resist deformation. It can also be conceptualized as the amount of energy that a gel can store.

A gel with a higher G' is considered a "firmer gel" and is ideal when there is a need for deep, targeted product deposition with less distribution of product into the surrounding tissues. However, because high G' products resist deformation, they may feel firmer within the tissues. Higher G' products are useful when structural definition, precision, or tissue lifting is needed. The G' is dependent on several factors, including the cross-linking density, the HA concentration, and the presence of unbound HA. Increasing cross-linking density and increasing HA concentration both increase G'.[6]

Table 2
Hyaluronic acid concentration of FDA-approved hyaluronic acid fillers

Product	HA Concentration (mg/mL)
Volbella	15
Vollure	17.5
Voluma	20
All Restylane products	20
Belotero Balance	22.5
RHA 2 RHA 3 RHA 4	23
Juvéderm Ultra Juvéderm Ultra Plus	24
Revanesse Versa	25

Some HA formulations contain lidocaine to alleviate the pain associated with injection. Adding lidocaine to HA gels seems to modify G′ and other gel properties.[20]

Gel viscosity
Gel viscosity is quantified by the viscous modulus, or G double prime (G″). G″ can be considered as a gel's resistance to dynamic forces and is also known as the loss modulus. A higher G″ gel is thicker and requires a greater extrusion force to be expressed through a needle (eg, peanut butter, rather than syrup).

G″ is a measure of a gel's ability to dissipate energy when force is applied, and this measure is reciprocally related to G′, the ability to store energy.

Together, G″ and G′ define the complex modulus, or G*, which represents a gel's total resistance to deformation, and is determined by the following formula:[21]

$$G^* = \sqrt{(G')^2 + (G'')^2}$$

Although fillers are viscoelastic, the elastic component is much more significant and the G′ value is much larger than that of G″. As such, G* and G′ are almost identical. G′ is more widely reported and considered a proxy for G*.

Elasticity and viscosity
Tan delta (δ) is a measure of a gel's balance of elasticity versus viscosity, and is defined by the ratio of G″ to G′.

$$\text{Tan } \delta = G''/G'$$

Gels characterized by a high tan δ, with values close to one, are predominantly viscous (eg, honey), whereas those characterized by a low tan delta, with values near zero, are predominantly elastic (eg, gelatin).

Table 3
Filler selection

Location	Filler
Tear trough	Restylane-L Belotero Balance
Midface	Restylane Lyft Juvéderm Voluma Restylane Contour RHA-4
Lips	Juvéderm Ultra Restylane Kysse Versa Lips Restylane Refyne
Nasolabial folds/marionette lines	RHA-3 Restylane Refyne Restylane Defyne Juvéderm Ultra Juvéderm Ultra Plus Juvéderm Vollure
Fine facial rhytids	Belotero Balance RHA-2
Liquid rhinoplasty	Restylane-L Restylane Lyft

There is no order of preference for the listed fillers.

FILLER SELECTION

No one product is optimal to achieve every single esthetic goal, and the rheologic properties described above must be considered when choosing the specific product and the injection tool. Consideration of all of these gel characteristics and rheologic measurements give the injector a sense of how this HA gel will behave in vivo. It is up to each injector to use this knowledge to choose the best gel to fit each area that they are choosing to inject. For example, when injecting an area such as the lips, one should choose a product that is not too firm and, depending on the patient's esthetic goals, either swells more or less. **Table 3** lists the authors' usual preferences for filler based on treatment location. There are other fillers that could be appropriate for specific indications that are not listed. In **Fig. 1**, the patient was treated with Restylane-L in the tear troughs and Restylane Lyft and Contour in the midface. Although both products support and volumize the midface, Restylane Contour is a softer gel and provides a more natural appearance in areas of movement. The patient in **Fig. 2** was treated

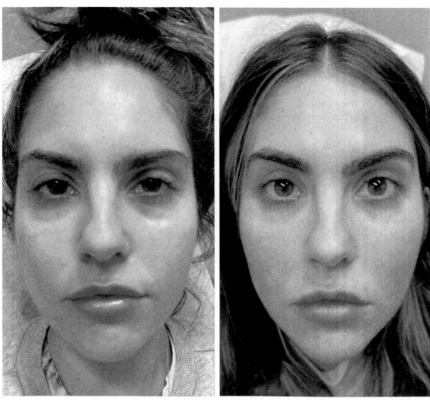

Fig. 1. Tear trough and midface filler. Restylane Contour and Lyft were used in the midface. Restylane-L was used in the tear troughs. (*Courtesy of* Sarah Taylor, RN/Bloom Facial Plastic Surgery.)

with Restylane-L in the nasal dorsum, which was chosen over Restylane Lyft for its smoothness and softness.

INJECTION CONSIDERATIONS AND ADVERSE EFFECTS

To safely obtain natural-looking results with dermal fillers, a thorough understanding of facial anatomy and appreciation for the patterns of change in the aging face are essential. Before injection, the prudent clinician considers the esthetic goal of the procedure, anesthesia, the product, depth and anatomic location of injection with special attention to possible complications, volume of product to be injected, the instrument to be used for injection (cannula vs needle), as well as the gauge of the instrument. Depth of injection in each anatomic area must be carefully considered given the risk of complications that include skin necrosis, vascular injury, filler embolization, and blindness.

With regard to anesthesia, some dermal filler products contain lidocaine, assisting with patient comfort while filling. Additional anesthetic, if used, is typically applied topically in a cream or gel form. Commonly used topical anesthetics

before dermal filler injection include compounded benzocaine–lidocaine–tetracaine, lidocaine–prilocaine, or one of these components alone.

Hyaluronidase is a naturally occurring enzyme that degrades HA and is a useful tool to reverse injected HA filler. Specifically, hyaluronidase can be used to eliminate inflammatory nodules, bumps, or superficially placed product. Most critically, it can treat vascular occlusion from intra-arterial injection.[22] When undesirable nodules or asymmetries occur postinjection, small doses of hyaluronidase can be used to dissolve the filler.[23] In the case of vascular occlusion, the recommended strategy is to Immediately flood the area with hyaluronidase, on the order of hundreds of units in order to quickly dissolve the filler and mitigate risks of skin necrosis and other tissue compromise.[24] Some providers will administer greater than 1000 units if large areas of skin are involved.[25] There is some controversy over how to treat vascular occlusion with visual compromise but due to the favorable risk–benefit ratio, retrobulbar injection of hyaluronidase is recommended if there is true vision loss.[25–28]

Related to the injection itself, side effects include pain, erythema, hematoma, and edema. These side effects are almost always minor and

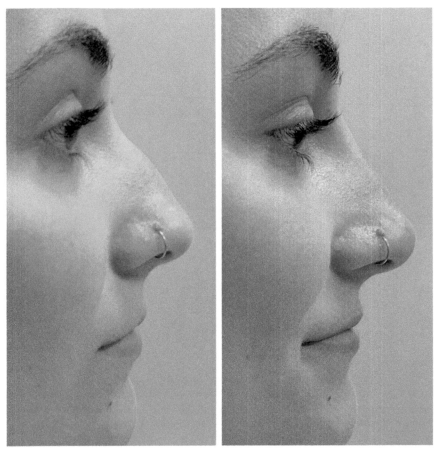

Fig. 2. Liquid rhinoplasty. Restylane-L was used cephalad to the dorsal hump to camouflage it. (*Courtesy of* Sarah Taylor, RN/Bloom Facial Plastic Surgery.)

self-resolving, necessitating only ice and compression for treatment.

Allergic reactions to HA filler additives—such as the cross-linker, BDDE, or lidocaine—are possible. Because chemical cross-linkers can be irritating and can incite a foreign body reaction in the skin, any residual active stabilizer must be removed from the product after the cross-linking process. Too much cross-linking may lead to biocompatibility issues, resulting in rejection, encapsulation, or delayed onset inflammatory events.

Delayed reactions include formation of foreign body granulomas, delayed onset swelling, or biofilms. After attempting to dissolve the product, these should be treated initially with antibiotics with further therapies, including oral or intralesional steroids or 5-fluorouracil, depending on response.[24]

FUTURE DIRECTIONS

A newer application of HA dermal filler products is skin boosting. Skin boosting refers to techniques used to enhance the appearance of aging skin. HA is administered via microdroplet injections into skin in an effort to provide the long-term hydration that topical products cannot achieve. There are currently no HA dermal filler products approved for the purpose of skin boosting in the US; however, there are products available in Europe, Canada, and Asia for this purpose. There is some limited evidence that these products can improve skin moisture, firmness, and glow.[29] There is also some evidence that the addition of skin boosting injections can enhance the results produced with botulinum toxin and conventional application of HA dermal filler.[30] Repeated treatments are usually necessary.

SUMMARY

HA is the most popular material to address volume loss and wrinkles associated with skin aging. Because HA is a naturally occurring component of the human skin, HA-derived fillers are well-suited for use in facial rejuvenation, are associated with a low risk of allergic reaction, and are long lasting.

The HA product can be reversed with injection of hyaluronidase to help mitigate any adverse events.

There are numerous HA dermal filler products available on the market, and these are differentiated by their physico-chemical characteristics and rheological properties. As the number of FDA-approved dermal filler products and approved indications for these products continues to increase, a basic understanding of these concepts is crucial to selecting the optimal filler for a particular situation.

CLINICS CARE POINTS

- Knowledge of physico-chemical characteristics and rheologic properties of hyaluronic acid (HA) dermal fillers is critical to choosing the right product for each patient.
- Degree of cross-linking, HA concentration, swelling factor, and G′ are highly relevant clinically. All injectors should understand these concepts.
- In-depth knowledge of vascular anatomy and proper injection technique are necessary to reduce the risk of adverse events.
- In the event of vascular occlusion, hyaluronidase needs to be injected immediately, in the range of a hundred units or more. Repeat injections may be necessary.

DISCLOSURE

Dr J.D. Bloom is a consultant, advisory board member, speaker's bureau member, trainer, and clinical investigator for Galderma and Allergan. He is also a consultant, advisory board member, speaker's bureau member and trainer for Revance Therapeutics and Endo Aesthetics.

REFERENCES

1. Lambros V. Observations on periorbital and midface aging. Plast Reconstr Surg 2007;120:1367–76.
2. Lambros V. Models of facial aging and implications for treatment. Clin Plast Surg 2008;35(3):319-317.
3. Rohrich RJ, Pessa JE. The fat compartments of the face: anatomy and clinical implications for cosmetic surgery. Plast Reconstr Surg 2007;119(7):2219–31.
4. Greco TM, Antunes MB, Yellin SA. Injectable fillers for volume replacement in the aging face. Facial Plast Surg 2012;28(1):8–20.
5. Sundaram H, Cassuto D. Biophysical characteristics of hyaluronic acid soft-tissue fillers and their relevance to aesthetic applications [published correction appears in Plast Reconstr Surg 2013 Nov;132(5):1378]. Plast Reconstr Surg 2013;132(4 Suppl 2):5S–21S.
6. Kablik J, Monheit GD, Yu L, et al. Comparative physical properties of hyaluronic acid dermal fillers. Dermatol Surg 2009;35(Suppl 1):302–12.
7. Global Hyaluronic Acid-based Dermal Fillers Market Report 2021: Market to Reach $5.8 Billion by 2027 - Single Phase Segment to Account for $3.3 Billion - ResearchAndMarkets.com" Business Wire. Available at: https://www.businesswire.com/news/home/20210507005262/en/Global-Hyaluronic-Acid-based-Dermal-Fillers-Market-Report-2021-Market-to-Reach-5.8-Billion-by-2027—Single-Phase-Segment-to-Account-for-3.3-Billion—ResearchAndMarkets.com. Accessed Oct 12, 2021.
8. Papakonstantinou E, Roth M, Karakiulakis G. Hyaluronic acid: a key molecule in skin aging. Dermatoendocrinol 2012;4(3):253–8.
9. Hascell V, Laurent T. Hyaluronan: structure and physical properties. Glycoforum: Hyaluronan Today; 1997. Available at: https://www.glycoforum.gr.jp/article/01A2.html. Accessed Sep 15, 2021.
10. Cockerham K, Hsu VJ. Collagen-based dermal fillers: past, present, and future. Facial Plast Surg 2009;25:106–13.
11. Restylane FDA approval letter. Available at: https://www.accessdata.fda.gov/cdrh_docs/pdf4/p040024a.pdf.
12. Sundaram H, Rohrich RJ, Liew S, et al. Cohesivity of hyaluronic acid fillers: development and clinical implications of a novel assay, pilot validation with a five-point grading scale, and evaluation of six U.S. Food and Drug Administration-approved fillers. Plast Reconstr Surg 2015;136(4):678–86.
13. Weissmann B, Meyer K. The structure of hyalobiuronic acid and of hyaluronic acid from umbilical cord. J Am Chem Soc 1954;76:1753–7.
14. Wang F, Garza LA, Kang S, et al. In vivo stimulation of de novo collagen production caused by cross-linked hyaluronic acid dermal filler injections in photodamaged human skin. Arch Dermatol 2007;143:155–63.
15. Landau M, Fagien S. Science of hyaluronic acid beyond filling: fibroblasts and their response to the extracellular matrix. Plast Reconstr Surg 2015;136(5 Suppl):188S–95S.
16. Liu L, Liu Y, Li J, et al. Microbial production of hyaluronic acid: current state, challenges, and perspectives. Microb Cell Fact 2011;10:99.
17. Tezel A, Fredrickson GH. The science of hyaluronic acid dermal fillers. J Cosmet Laser Ther 2008;10:35–42.
18. Beasley KL, Weiss MA, Weiss RA. Hyaluronic acid fillers: A comprehensive review. Facial Plast Surg 2009;25(2):86–94.
19. Sutherland IW. Novel and established applications of microbial polysaccharides. Trends Biotechnol 1998;16:41–6.

20. Micheels P, Eng MO. Rheological properties of several hyaluronic acid-based gels: a comparative study. J Drugs Dermatol 2018;17(9):948–54.

21. Pierre S, Liew S, Bernardin A. Basics of dermal filler rheology. Dermatol Surg 2015;41(Suppl 1):S120–6.

22. Cavallini M, Gazzola R, Metalla M, et al. The role of hyaluronidase in the treatment of complications from hyaluronic acid dermal fillers. Aesthet Surg J 2013;33(8):1167–74.

23. Alam M, Hughart R, Geisler A, et al. Effectiveness of low doses of hyaluronidase to remove hyaluronic acid filler nodules. A randomized clinical trial. JAMA Dermatol 2018;154(7):765–72.

24. Jones DH, Fitzgerald R, Cox SE, et al. Preventing and treating adverse events of injectable fillers: Evidence-based recommendations from the American Society for Dermatologic Surgery multidisciplinary task force. Dermatol Surg 2021;47(2):214–26.

25. DeLorenzi C. New high dose pulused hyaluronidase protocol for hyaluronic acid filler vascular adverse events. Aesthet Surg J 2017;37(7):814–25.

26. Carruthers JDA, Fagien S, Rohrich RJ, et al. Blindness caused by cosmetic filler injection: a review of cause and therapy. Plast Reconstr Surg 2014;134:1197–201.

27. King M, Convery C, Davies E. This month's guideline: the use of hyaluronidase in aesthetic practice (v2.4). J Clin Aesthet Dermatol 2018;11(6):E61–8.

28. Philipp-Dormston WG, Bergfeld D, Sommer BM, et al. Consensus statement on prevention and management of adverse effects following rejuvenation procedures with hyaluronic acid-based fillers. J Eur Acad Dermatol Venereol 2017;31:1088–95.

29. Ayatollahi A, Firooz A, Samadi A. Evaluation of safety and efficacy of booster injections of hyaluronic acid in improving the facial skin quality. J Cosmet Dermatol 2020;19:2267–72.

30. Cartier H, Hedén P, Delmar H, et al. Repeated full-face aesthetic combination treatment with abobotulinumtoxinA, hyaluronic acid filler, and skin-boosting hyaluronic acid after monotherapy with abobotulinumtoxinA or hyaluronic acid filler. Dermatol Surg 2020;46(4):475–82.

Treatment of Periorbital Vascularity, Erythema, and Hyperpigmentation

Christen B. Samaan, MD[a], Todd V. Cartee, MD[a],*

KEYWORDS

- Periorbital hyperpigmentation • Classification • Lightening topical • Chemical peel • Laser
- Blepharoplasty

KEY POINTS

Periorbital hyperpigmentation (POH) is often multifactorial and impacts patient's emotional well-being and overall quality of life.

- POH can be classified into pigmented, vascular, structural, and mixed subtypes.
- Etiology of POH should be taken into consideration when forming a management plan.
- Treatment varies from topical therapy, chemical peels, dermal fillers, platelet-rich plasma, lasers, to blepharoplasty.

INTRODUCTION

Periorbital discoloration or periorbital hyperpigmentation (POH) is a very frequent presenting complaint of patients. It can affect the individual in many ways because of its perception as a sign of aging, appearing fatigued, and overall negative impact on quality of life (QOL). POH presents as a light to dark brown pigmentation or violaceous discoloration involving the upper and/or lower eyelids. Clinical presentation depends on the etiology and skin color of the patient. Diagnosis is made based on history and clinical examination.

Despite being a common chief complaint, POH is an ill-defined concept. Incidence and prevalence are difficult to estimate due to underreporting of the presentation. Studies are predominantly focused on Asian populations. Based on these studies, POH occurs more frequently in patients with skin of color (SOC) and women.[1]

CLASSIFICATION

The cause of POH is often multifactorial and having a better understanding of the etiology can enhance treatment success. Classification of POH can be divided into vascular, structural, pigmented, and mixed subtypes (**Fig. 1**).[2]

- *Vascular*. The vascular subtype of POH is due to the superficial location of vasculature or thin skin overlying the orbicularis oculi muscle (**Table 1**). **Fig. 2** shows an example of prominent periorbital veins contributing to a mixed vascular and structural POH. The vascular subtype can also be associated with periorbital edema.
- *Structural*. Abnormalities in the periorbital surface contours lead to structural shadows and the appearance of POH (**Fig. 3**). Orbital fat pseudoherniation, skin laxity, tear trough depression, or periorbital edema is the causes of the structural subtype (see **Table 1**).

Conflict of Interest: The authors have no potential conflicts of interest to disclose.
[a] Department of Dermatology, Penn State Health, Milton S. Hershey Medical Center, 500 University Drive, HU 14, Hershey, PA 17033, USA
* Corresponding author.
E-mail address: tcartee@pennstatehealth.psu.edu

Facial Plast Surg Clin N Am 30 (2022) 309–319
https://doi.org/10.1016/j.fsc.2022.03.005

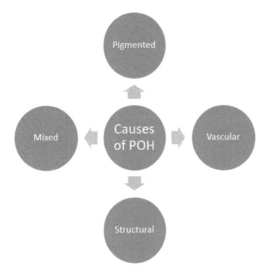

Fig. 1. Classification of POH.

- *Pigmented*. The pigmented subtype is due to increased melanin in the dermis or epidermis. Causative factors of pigmented subtype vary from genetics (**Fig. 4**), extension of pigmentary demarcation lines, nevus of Ota or Hori, dermatitis, postinflammatory hyperpigmentation (PIH), or drug induced (see **Table 1**).[2]

EVALUATION

Differentiating between the different subtypes of POH can be challenging as multiple contributing factors can be present. Manual stretching of the

Table 1
Etiologies of POH. PIH: Postinflammatory hyperpigmentation

POH Type	Causes
Pigmented	Genetics
	PIH
	Extension of demarcation lines
	Nevus of Ota
	Nevus of Hori
	Drug induced
	Atopic or allergic contact dermatitis
Vascular	Superficial location of vasculature
	Thin overlying skin
Structural	Pseudoherniation of orbital fat pads
	Skin laxity
	Photodamage
	Periorbital edema

lower eyelid during the physical examination can help elucidate the subtype by differentiating between true pigment depositions, superficial vasculature, or shadowing effect (**Table 2**).[3]

Clinical pearls for physical examination:
1. First, evaluate discoloration with direct lighting:
   a. In the structural subtype, discoloration improves or disappears with direct lighting
2. Second, manually stretch the lower eyelid:
   a. An increase in the violaceous color indicates vasculature subtype (see **Fig. 3**)
   b. True pigment deposit would not result in any change in color (see **Fig. 4**)
   c. Structural subtype improves with manual stretching as the shadowing effect is eliminated (see **Fig. 3**)

Dermoscopy can be helpful in making the important distinction between vascular and pigmented subtypes. **Fig. 5** shows an exaggerated reticular pigment network, characteristic of melanin deposition in basal keratinocytes or at the dermoepidermal junction along rete ridges. This is a common pattern in pigmented POH. There are fine facial blood vessels near the lash line but this patient's POH is predominantly pigmented.

TREATMENT
Topical therapy

Topical treatments are commonly used as they are readily accessible (**Table 3**). Regimens for POH are often extrapolated from studies based on the treatment of melasma and other disorders of hyperpigmentation. An understanding of key ingredients in products targeting POH can help physicians determine optimum therapy based on the etiology.

Hydroquinone is the most widely used skin lightening agent for pigmented subtype POH, though it has not been studied as either monotherapy or in combination with a topical retinoid for this indication. Hydroquinone targets hyperpigmentation by inhibiting the tyrosinase enzyme and thus inhibiting the conversion of dopamine to melanin. Retinoids play a role in promoting keratinocyte proliferation and epidermal turnover and are hypothesized to reduce tyrosinase expression.[4] Irritation is a common side effect as hydroquinone can be difficult to tolerate on eyelids, especially in combination with a topical retinoid.

Other topical treatments include kojic acid, arbutin, azelaic acid, resveratrol, vitamin K, and caffeine pads. Azelaic acid can be considered in the setting of postinflammatory hyperpigmentation

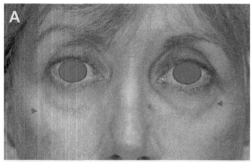

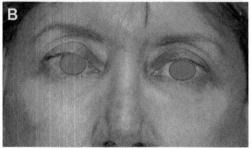

Fig. 2. (*A*) Mixed vascular and structural POH; (*B*) status post–long-pulsed Nd:YAG laser for periorbital veins and dermal filler into tear troughs and palpebromalar grooves. Her prominent preprocedural reticular veins are indicated by blue arrows which resolved after 2 laser treatments.

(PIH). Arbutin should be used with caution as the topical treatment can paradoxically cause hyperpigmentation at high doses.[5] One study showed improvement in POH, skin elasticity, and appearance of hydration when vitamin K and caffeine were applied simultaneously compared with placebo in a split-face, single-blinded trial.[6] Resveratrol exhibited 19% improvement in dermal thickness in one study of periorbital skin.[7]

Vitamin C is hypothesized to improve POH, especially vascular subtype, by promoting collagen production to increase dermal thickness.[8] Placebo-controlled trials of topical Vitamin C for this specific indication are lacking. Although it is hypothesized that topical ascorbic acid also inhibits melanogenesis, one placebo-controlled trial did not show significant improvement in melanin content.[8]

Chemical peels

Chemical peels are commonly used to treat various causes of hyperpigmentation. Special considerations should be taken when treating patients with Fitzpatrick skin type IV–VI due to increased risk of PIH. Pretreating with topical retinoid and hydroquinone reduces the risk of PIH and may improve the appearance of POH given their mechanism of action. Pretreating with topical

retinoid may also accelerate healing and thus improve downtime and patient satisfaction.[9] Topical retinoid and hydroquinone are generally discontinued 48 hours before the peel although a longer period is required if they are inducing any irritation.

One study included patients with Fitzpatrick skin types II–IV who underwent a chemical peel for the treatment of POH weekly for a total of 4 sessions with 15% lactic acid (LA) and 3.75% trichloroacetic acid (TCA).[10] The regimen resulted in significant aesthetic improvement in almost all the patients. The authors note that the aesthetic outcome remained for at least 4 to 6 months on follow-up when appropriate sun protection was used.[10]

A study by Dayal and colleagues[11] showed that 20% glycolic acid (GA) and 15% LA peel are more effective than topical vitamin C in treating mixed subtype POH. Adverse effects were reported at higher rate in the GA group and included erythema, burning sensation, irritation, dryness, and telangiectasia. Given the current findings in the literature, ascorbic acid is not recommended as monotherapy for pigmented or mixed subtype POH.

Patient's skin type and subtype of POH should be taken into consideration when selecting the depth of peel. Superficial chemical peels, such as 15% LA, 3.75% TCA, and 20% GA, are appropriate and safe for use in patients with SOC to treat the pigmented subtype of POH. The structural subtype requires a medium depth chemical peel.[12] In Fitzpatrick I–III skin, a medium depth chemical peel, such as 35% TCA or a Jessner's and TCA combination, can be applied for the treatment of periorbital rhytids and photodamage.

Lasers

Lasers are becoming increasingly integrated into treatment plans for POH. A systematic review of 10 studies (n = 143) found that 81.2% of participants had a good to excellent response to laser therapy for POH.[13] However, one of the difficulties in fully assessing the efficacy of treatment with laser therapy is that most of the studies are not based on the classification of POH or skin type. In addition to the lack of randomized controlled trials, studies vary in assessing response to treatment and time points at which the data are obtained. Despite the paucity of data, currently published studies have shown that lasers can be effective, safe, and provide satisfactory results with long-term positive outcomes when used appropriately.[13]

- *Vascular*. Facial telangiectasias are most commonly treated with pulse dye laser

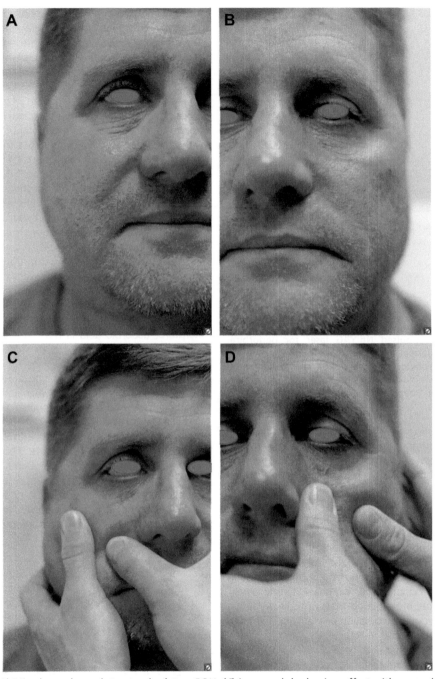

Fig. 3. (*A, B*) Mixed vascular and structural subtype POH; (*C*) improved shadowing effect with manual stretching of lower eyelid; (*D*) mild improvement of shadowing effect but increased prominence of periorbital reticular veins.

(PDL), potassium titanyl phosphate (KTP) laser, and intense pulse light (IPL).[14] Unlike facial telangiectasias, reticular veins are larger (1–3 mm), located deeper, and are commonly seen on the lower eyelids, infraorbital cheeks, and temples. Reticular veins can significantly contribute to vascular POH, creating a bluish hue across the lower lid. Due to their depth, deeper penetrating long-pulsed Nd:YAG is a more effective treatment of reticular veins than the aforementioned vascular lasers.[15] A study by Lai and Goldman[16] reported nearly

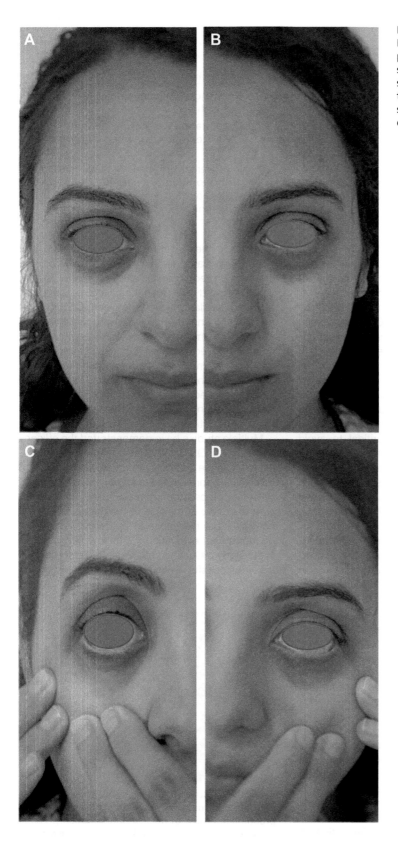

Fig. 4. (*A, B*) Pigmented subtype POH; (*C, D*) appearance of pigmentation unchanged to slightly improved on manual stretching of lower eyelid. Patient's POH mostly pigmented subtype with mild shadowing due to periorbital edema.

Table 2
Clinical presentation and physician exam findings of POH

POH Type	Clinical Presentation	Examination
Pigmented	Patches of brown to gray discoloration	No change in pigment intensity on manual stretching
Vascular	Blue to violaceous discoloration mainly involving the lower eyelid with possible visible veins	Discoloration worsens, seems more violaceous in color when skin stretched
Structural	Eye bags, gray shadow, or hollow appearance especially in the medial inferior periorbital region	Improvement of shadows/appearance of discoloration when eyelid stretched. No discoloration present with direct lighting.

a 100% improvement of periocular reticular veins after treatment with dynamically cooled, variable spot size 1064 nm Nd:YAG. Similar results at the time of treatment and at 12-months follow-up were seen in a study by Ma and colleagues[17] in 26 Chinese women with Fitzpatrick skin type III and IV. Most patients require 1 to 2 sessions and treatment parameters are dependent on the size of the veins as higher energy may be needed for full-thickness penetration into the vessel.[15–17] Generally, a longer pulse duration varying from 20 to 50 ms, nonoverlapping pulses, and epidermal cooling are critical to avoid thermal injury to the epidermis.[15–17] Long-pulsed Nd:YAG is associated with a lower risk of pigmentary side effects and is safer in darker skin types as there is decreased melanin absorption at the 1064 nm wavelength.[18]

- *Pigmented.* For targeting the pigmented subtype, a few studies have looked at Q-switched lasers (QSL), either as monotherapy or in combination with other interventions. QSL, such as QS Ruby (694 nm), QS Alexandrite (755 nm), and QS Nd:YAG (1064 nm), treat pigmentary lesions through selective photothermolysis of targeted melanosomes.[19] In a study by Watanabe and colleagues,[20] 8 Japanese patients with biopsy-proven dermal melanocytosis on the lower eyelids were treated with QS 694 nm wavelength with a fluence of 6.0 to 7.0 J/cm^2 over 1 to 5 sessions. Patients treated with more than one session reported good to excellent response and side effects localized to the treated area resolved within a week.[20] A study by Lowe and colleagues[21] reported greater than 50% improvement of POH in 90% of the subjects that were treated with QS 694 nm and noted a decrease of dermal melanin deposition on posttreatment histologic evaluation.[21]

Fewer studies exist to evaluate the efficacy of QS 755 nm laser in the treatment of POH, but one would predict similar efficacy. A prospective, split-face study by Rosenbach and colleagues[22] reported similar efficacy between QS 755 nm and QS 1064 nm laser in improving hyperpigmentation. The melanin reflectance spectrometry score improved after the first session and significant clinical improvement was noted after 3 sessions. Both the QS 755 nm and QS 1064 nm lasers resulted in a significant reduction of epidermal pigmentation and melanocytes on histologic evaluation.[22]

Multiple studies have demonstrated the efficacy and safety of QS Nd:YAG laser in treating POH using low fluence and pulse duration.[22,23] In addition to clinical improvement and patient satisfaction, reflectance spectrophotometer showed a significant decrease of melanin in the upper dermis but no significant difference in epidermal melanin in posttreatment evaluation.[23] The low fluence used in the study by Xu and colleagues[23] is extrapolated from successful treatment of other pigmented

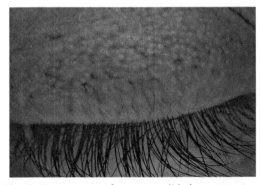

Fig. 5. Dermoscopy of upper eyelid shows exaggerated pigment network with a reticular pattern (the predominant cause of the POH in this patient). Visible veins are also located inferiorly but not in the areas of POH.

Table 3
Treatment modalities for consideration based on POH subtype

POH Type	Causes	Treatment Options
Pigmented	Genetics Extension of demarcation lines Nevus of Ota Nevus of Hori	Hydroquinone Retinoid Kojic acid Azelaic acid Vitamin K + caffeine Arbutin Chemical peel Q switched or picosecond lasers
	Drug induced PIH Dermatitis	+ Stop offending medication Treat underlying condition
Vascular	Superficial vasculature	PDL Long pulsed Nd:YAG Vitamin C Carboxytherapy
	Thin skin overlying orbicularis oculi muscle	Injectable filler PRP
Structural	Skin laxity	Chemical peel (superficial or medium depth) Fractional laser resurfacing (ablative or nonablative)
	Orbital fat pad pseudoherniation	Blepharoplasty
	Tear trough deformity	Filler (HA, fat, calcium hydroxylapatite) Blepharoplasty
	Periorbital edema	Treat underlying cause

Abbreviations: PIH, Postinflammatory hyperpigmentation; PDL, Pulsed dye laser; PRP, Platelet-rich plasma

disorders with QS Nd:YAG. The pulse width of the QS Nd:YAG is not sufficient to engender vasospasm in vessels; however, some improvement of the erythema index can be noted if present along with pigmentation.[23]

A new emerging therapy for the treatment of pigmentary disorders is the picosecond laser.[24–26] A retrospective study by Levin and colleagues[27] showed comparable improvement of pigmented lesions, side effects, and patient satisfaction between the QSL group and 755 nm alexandrite picosecond laser in patients with Fitzpatrick skin types III–VI. The picosecond 755 nm laser has been shown to be effective and safe in patients with Fitzpatrick skin type IV to VI with transient side effects resolving within weeks of treatment.[24–27] One small study showed promise using picosecond lasers specifically for POH.[28] More research is needed but this newer therapy may be an effective and safe option for all skin types with lower risk of PIH due to lower photothermal damage.[25]

- *Structural.* Ablative and nonablative laser resurfacing are frequently used to improve skin texture and are often used in the treatment

of POH, especially structural subtype. Fully ablative CO_2 laser resurfacing resulted in 50% clinical improvement after 9 weeks in a study by West and Alster.[29] However, there was no significant improvement in melanin measurements obtained using a handheld reflectance spectrometer pre and posttreatment.[29] Postoperative PIH was reported in 33% of patients and lasted for 12 weeks.[29] Similar results were seen in a study of 67 patients with upper eyelid dermatochalasis and periorbital rhytids with significant improvement after treatment with traditional CO_2 laser.[30]

Ablative fractional resurfacing with a CO_2 laser also improves deep wrinkles and textural irregularities but with considerably less downtime and fewer risks than traditional ablative laser.[31] Nonablative fractional laser spares the overlying epidermis, leading to more rapid healing and less downtime than traditional and fractional ablative laser resurfacing.[32] The fractionated 1550 nm erbium-doped fiber laser has been reported in the literature to improve the pigmented POH subtype at 4-week intervals over 4 months.[32] A recent study by Horovitz and colleagues[33] reported a significant improvement of wrinkles based on physician assessment after treatment with 1565 nm Er:glass fiber laser. Although patients reported a mild-moderate improvement 8 weeks after treatment, minimal side effects and downtime were noted.[33] Physicians should discuss with patients that improvement from nonablative fractional lasers can progress over 6 months.[33] Furthermore, studies have generally supported the safety of nonablative fractional lasers in SOC.[34] However, these studies contained very few subjects with Fitzpatrick V or VI skin type so caution and conservative treatment parameters are advised.[34]

When lasers are being considered to treat POH, the possibility of PIH should be discussed with the patient. Patient counseling when using lasers in the periocular region includes appropriate protective eyewear. When feasible, targeted skin should be stretched outside the orbital rim and laser beams should be angled away from the orbit. The authors usually use metal corneal eye shields when performing laser inside the bony orbital rim.[14]

Filler

Fillers can be an effective treatment for the the structural subtype by eliminating shadows formed from tear trough depression, by subcutaneous fat loss or fat pad descent, or from overlying skin thinning. Fillers are not a substitute for surgical correction in the presence of significant orbital fat prolapse. Treatment with fillers includes hyaluronic acid (HA), calcium hydroxylapatite, and autologous fat grafts.

Small volumes of low G′, relatively thin HA fillers are most commonly used for tear trough correction and are injected into the tear trough deformity with a needle or cannula at the supraperiosteal plane, ideally deep to the orbicularis oculi muscle. More recently, a subdermal, microdroplet placement of low molecular weight HA filler has been proposed.[35] This injection method is not recommended for patients with global volume loss and significant eyelid skin laxity as it may produce eyelid or malar edema.[35]

Fat grafts are another treatment modality for structural subtype POH or translucent lower eyelid skin resulting in increased vascularity and visible orbicularis oculi muscle. Another advantage of autologous fat transplant is decreased risk of blue cast or Tyndall effect caused by the superficial placement of HA filler. However, visible fat lumps can occur resulting in poor cosmetic outcomes. Collagenase-digested fat cell grafts placed in the dermal layer can improve lower eyelid contouring while decreasing the risk of visible collections of fat.[36]

Patients with significant tear trough deformity, including postseptal fat pad pseudoherniation and redundant lower eyelid skin, may not benefit from soft tissue filler. The risk of adverse events when using volume augmentation with filler, such as Tyndall effect and blindness, should be discussed with the patient. Although the risk of intravascular occlusion events is very low with either needles or cannulas, injection with microcannula is associated with a lower risk.[37] Overall, the risk of occlusion with needle injection decreases with experience and whether a needle or cannula is appropriate ultimately depends on the patient, anatomic site, and pathology being treated.[37]

Other injectable

Platelet-rich plasma (PRP) injections decrease the visibility of underlying muscles and vasculature by increasing the thickness of the epidermis and dermis. Mehryan and colleagues[38] treated 10 patients in a single session with intradermal injections of 1.5 mL PRP into the nasojugal groove and crow's feet region. Injection of PRP resulted in significant improvement of infraorbital color homogeneity with 80% of patients achieving fair to good improvement after 3 months.[38] Although PRP has been shown to increase the thickness of the epidermis and dermis, it is not associated with significant improvement in melanin content, stratum corneum hydration, or wrinkle volume.[38] Most common side effects associated with PRP include mild/transient pain and ecchymosis that can last 1 to 2 weeks. These side effects can be minimized by using a cannula.

Although the mechanism of action of carboxytherapy is unclear, one study has shown that subcutaneous CO_2 injection once a week for several weeks resulted in improvement in fine wrinkles and overall POH.[39] Carboxytherapy was slightly more effective and associated with less adverse events when injected in the periorbital region in patients with pigmented, vascular, and mixed-type POH.[39]

Surgery

Blepharoplasty should be considered in patients with advanced structural subtype POH, who possess significant lower eyelid skin laxity combined with orbital fat pad pseudoherniation. Blepharoplasty can improve POH by decreasing the shadowing effect by restoring the normal anatomy and contouring of the periorbital region and removing excess skin. For complex cases, a

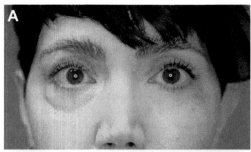

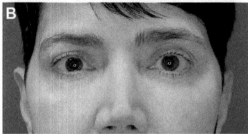

Fig. 6. (A) Patient with a history of prior direct trans-cutaneous lower eyelid fat pad resection greater than 10 years ago and inappropriately placed hyaluronic acid filler combined with prominent infraorbital reticular veins and telangiectasias. She underwent hyaluronidase injections to reverse her filler followed by 3 sessions of laser (KTP and Nd:YAG) to lower eyelids for the prominent vasculature. She then underwent revision transconjunctival bilateral lower eyelid blepharoplasty with abdominal fat transfer. (B). Patient 2.5 months postop. (Photos courtesy of Jessyka G. Lighthall, MD.)

multifaceted approach may be used to optimize patient outcomes (Fig. 6).

DISCUSSION

Various treatment modalities have been studied to improve the appearance of POH in patients (see Table 3). As discussed above, identifying the underlying etiology is crucial for effective treatment. In addition, taking into consideration the patient's skin type is important as it can impact the efficacy and safety of certain interventions.

- *Pigmented.* Pigmented subtype POH is due to melanin deposition in the epidermal or dermal layer. Treatment is aimed at reducing the melanin content.
  - For any skin type, bleaching agents such as hydroquinone and kojic acid as monotherapy or in combination with a topical retinoid are commonly prescribed as first-line therapy. Although hydroquinone is widely used, there are limited studies evaluating its efficacy and safety in the periocular region.

- Superficial chemical peels can be added if a patient is not responding within 2 to 3 months of topical therapy and should be repeated for 3 to 4 sessions. In patients with SOC, superficial peels can be safely used and the area treated with chemical peel should be extended to include the entire face.[10,11] All patients can be pre-treated with topical hydroquinone and retinoid if they are not already on this treatment.[9]
  - Lasers can be used in patients with significant periorbital melanosis or in patients who are not responding to topical therapies alone. Q-switched lasers are effective in eliminating pigment. Picosecond lasers offer a new therapeutic option with potentially increased efficacy and more safety for patients with SOC, but more studies are needed for use in POH.[27,28]
- *Vascular.* Vascular subtype POH can be due to the superficial location of vasculature or thin skin overlying the orbicularis oculi muscle.
  - Laser therapy is the most effective intervention in vascular subtype POH.
  - Lasers emitting shorter wavelengths, such as PDL and KTP are used to target facial telangiectasia.[14] For patients with prominent reticular veins as a component of their POH, long-pulsed Nd:YAG has been proven effective in 3 studies and is a reliable intervention in the authors' hands (see Fig. 2). In patients with darker skin color, Nd:YAG is recommended due to minimal interaction with epidermal melanin.[17,18]
  - Vitamin C can be added to the treatment plan or used as monotherapy for patients not amenable to laser intervention. Although not commonly considered first-line therapy, carboxytherapy can be used as adjunct therapy if the vascular component of POH is nonresponsive to topical and laser therapy.
  - Injectable filler and PRP are recommended for POH due to thin skin overlying muscle and vasculature. Subcutaneous PRP injection can be effective but its use is limited by the lack of tolerance to prolonged ecchymosis by patients. The authors usually can avoid this by using a cannula for injection.
- *Structural.* Mid-facial descent, tear trough deformity, and skin laxity cause a shadowing effect in the periorbital region.
  - Medium depth chemical peels can be trialed initially if photoaging is mild in patients with lighter skin color. Fractional ablative laser resurfacing is the authors' treatment

of choice for improving more advanced dermatochalasis and textural irregularities of the periorbital skin. Ablative lasers have increased risk of PIH and prolonged recovery periods in SOC. Nonablative fractional laser resurfacing is preferred in patients with SOC although more treatments are required.[30,34]

- Filler is first-line therapy for tear trough deformity (see **Fig. 2**).
- Blepharoplasty should be considered for the treatment of pronounced orbital fat pad pseudoherniation.

SUMMARY

POH is a common concern for patients due to its effect on a patient's well-being and negative impact on QOL. A number of treatment modalities exist for POH varying from over-the-counter topical treatments to surgery. Unfortunately, data from randomized controlled trials on the efficacy and safety of these interventions in POH are limited. However, successful strategies for improving POH do exist. As each treatment modality has different targets, care should be taken to identify causative factors and classification of POH. As the etiology of POH is often multifactorial, a combination of treatment options may be necessary.

REFERENCES

1. Sheth PB, Shah HA, Dave JN. Periorbital hyperpigmentation: a study of its prevalence, common causative factors and its association with personal habits and other disorders. Indian J Dermatol 2014;59(2): 151–7.
2. Huang YL, Chang SL, Ma L, et al. Clinical analysis and classification of dark eye circle. Int J Dermatol 2014;53(2):164–70.
3. Sarkar R, Ranjan R, Garg S, et al. Periorbital hyperpigmentation: a comprehensive review. J Clin Aesthet Dermatol 2016;9(1):49–55.
4. Sato K, Morita M, Ichikawa C, et al. Depigmenting mechanisms of all-trans retinoic acid and retinol on B16 melanoma cells. Biosci Biotechnol Biochem 2008;72(10):2589–97.
5. Ertam I, Mutlu B, Unal I, et al. Efficiency of ellagic acid and arbutin in melasma: a randomized, prospective, open-label study. J Dermatol 2008;35(9): 570–4.
6. Ahmadraji F, Shatalebi MA. Evaluation of the clinical efficacy and safety of an eye counter pad containing caffeine and vitamin K in emulsified Emu oil base. Adv Biomed Res 2015;4:10.
7. Farris P, Yatskayer M, Chen N, et al. Evaluation of efficacy and tolerance of a nighttime topical antioxidant containing resveratrol, baicalin, and vitamin e for treatment of mild to moderately photodamaged skin. J Drugs Dermatol 2014;13(12):1467–72.
8. Ohshima H, Mizukoshi K, Oyobikawa M, et al. Effects of vitamin C on dark circles of the lower eyelids: quantitative evaluation using image analysis and echogram. Skin Res Technol 2009;15(2):214–7.
9. Hevia O, Nemeth AJ, Taylor JR. Tretinoin accelerates healing after trichloroacetic acid chemical peel. Arch Dermatol 1991;127(5):678–82.
10. Vavouli C, Katsambas A, Gregoriou S, et al. Chemical peeling with trichloroacetic acid and lactic acid for infraorbital dark circles. J Cosmet Dermatol 2013;12(3):204–9.
11. Dayal S, Sahu P, Jain VK, et al. Clinical efficacy and safety of 20% glycolic peel, 15% lactic peel, and topical 20% vitamin C in constitutional type of periorbital melanosis: a comparative study. J Cosmet Dermatol 2016;15(4):367–73.
12. Manaloto RM, Alster TS. Periorbital rejuvenation: a review of dermatologic treatments. Dermatol Surg 1999;25(1):1–9.
13. Roohaninasab M, Sadeghzadeh-Bazargan A, Goodarzi A. Effects of laser therapy on periorbital hyperpigmentation: a systematic review on current studies. Lasers Med Sci 2021;36(9):1781–9.
14. Hiscox B, Wu WJ, Markus RF. Advanced laser therapy for cutaneous vascular lesions of the eyelid and face. 2016:
15. Lee TS, Kwek JWM, Ellis DAF. Treatment of periocular and temporal reticular veins with 1064-nm Nd: YAG Laser. J Cosmet Dermatol 2020;19(9):2306–12.
16. Lai SW, Goldman MP. Treatment of facial reticular veins with dynamically cooled, variable spot-sized 1064 nm Nd:YAG laser. J Cosmet Dermatol 2007; 6(1):6–8.
17. Ma G, Lin XX, Hu XJ, et al. Treatment of venous infraorbital dark circles using a long-pulsed 1,064-nm neodymium-doped yttrium aluminum garnet laser. Dermatol Surg 2012;38(8):1277–82.
18. Sherwood KA, Murray S, Kurban AK, et al. Effect of wavelength on cutaneous pigment using pulsed irradiation. J Invest Dermatol 1989;92(5):717–20.
19. Anderson RR, Margolis RJ, Watenabe S, et al. Selective photothermolysis of cutaneous pigmentation by Q-switched Nd: YAG laser pulses at 1064, 532, and 355 nm. J Invest Dermatol 1989;93(1):28–32.
20. Watanabe S, Nakai K, Ohnishi T. Condition known as "dark rings under the eyes" in the Japanese population is a kind of dermal melanocytosis which can be successfully treated by Q-switched ruby laser. Dermatol Surg 2006;32(6):785–9 [discussion: 789].
21. Lowe NJ, Wieder JM, Shorr N, et al. Infraorbital pigmented skin. Preliminary observations of laser therapy. Dermatol Surg 1995;21(9):767–70.

22. Rosenbach A, Williams CM, Alster TS. Comparison of the Q-switched alexandrite (755 nm) and Q-switched Nd:YAG (1064 nm) lasers in the treatment of benign melanocytic nevi. Dermatol Surg 1997;23(4):239–44 [discussion: 244-5].

23. Xu TH, Yang ZH, Li YH, et al. Treatment of infraorbital dark circles using a low-fluence Q-switched 1,064-nm laser. Dermatol Surg 2011;37(6):797–803.

24. Chan JC, Shek SY, Kono T, et al. A retrospective analysis on the management of pigmented lesions using a picosecond 755-nm alexandrite laser in Asians. Lasers Surg Med 2016;48(1):23–9.

25. Haimovic A, Brauer JA, Cindy Bae Y-S, et al. Safety of a picosecond laser with diffractive lens array (DLA) in the treatment of Fitzpatrick skin types IV to VI: A retrospective review. J Am Acad Dermatol 2016;74(5):931–6.

26. Kung KY, Shek SY, Yeung CK, et al. Evaluation of the safety and efficacy of the dual wavelength picosecond laser for the treatment of benign pigmented lesions in Asians. Lasers Surg Med 2019;51(1):14–22.

27. Levin MK, Ng E, Bae YS, et al. Treatment of pigmentary disorders in patients with skin of color with a novel 755 nm picosecond, Q-switched ruby, and Q-switched Nd:YAG nanosecond lasers: A retrospective photographic review. Lasers Surg Med 2016;48(2):181–7.

28. Vanaman Wilson MJ, Jones IT, Bolton J, et al. Prospective studies of the efficacy and safety of the picosecond 755, 1,064, and 532 nm lasers for the treatment of infraorbital dark circles. Lasers Surg Med 2018;50(1):45–50.

29. West TB, Alster TS. Improvement of infraorbital hyperpigmentation following carbon dioxide laser resurfacing. Dermatol Surg 1998;24(6):615–6.

30. Alster TS, Bellew SG. Improvement of dermatochalasis and periorbital rhytides with a high-energy pulsed CO2 laser: a retrospective study. Dermatol Surg 2004;30(4 Pt 1):483–7 [discussion: 487].

31. Tierney EP, Hanke CW, Watkins L. Treatment of lower eyelid rhytids and laxity with ablative fractionated carbon-dioxide laser resurfacing: Case series and review of the literature. J Am Acad Dermatol 2011;64(4):730–40.

32. Moody MN, Landau JM, Goldberg LH, et al. Fractionated 1550-nm erbium-doped fiber laser for the treatment of periorbital hyperpigmentation. Dermatol Surg 2012;38(1):139–42.

33. Horovitz T, Clementoni MT, Artzi O. Nonablative laser skin resurfacing for periorbital wrinkling-A case series of 16 patients. J Cosmet Dermatol 2021;20(1):99–104.

34. Kaushik SB, Alexis AF. Nonablative Fractional Laser Resurfacing in Skin of Color: Evidence-based Review. J Clin Aesthet Dermatol 2017;10(6):51–67.

35. Shah-Desai S, Joganathan V. Novel technique of non-surgical rejuvenation of infraorbital dark circles. J Cosmet Dermatol 2021;20(4):1214–20.

36. Youn S, Shin JI, Kim JD, et al. Correction of infraorbital dark circles using collagenase-digested fat cell grafts. Dermatol Surg 2013;39(5):766–72.

37. Alam M, Kakar R, Dover JS, et al. Rates of Vascular Occlusion Associated With Using Needles vs Cannulas for Filler Injection. JAMA Dermatol 2021;157(2):174–80.

38. Mehryan P, Zartab H, Rajabi A, et al. Assessment of efficacy of platelet-rich plasma (PRP) on infraorbital dark circles and crow's feet wrinkles. J Cosmet Dermatol 2014;13(1):72–8.

39. Nofal E, Elkot R, Nofal A, et al. Evaluation of carboxytherapy and platelet-rich plasma in treatment of periorbital hyperpigmentation: A comparative clinical trial. J Cosmet Dermatol 2018;17(6):1000–7.

Advances in Nonsurgical Periocular Rejuvenation

Jeffrey Desmond Markey, MD[a],*, William Matthew White, MD[b]

KEYWORDS

- Tear trough • Periocular • Hyaluronic acid • Platelet-rich plasma • Calcium hydroxyapatite
- Poly-L-lactic acid • Injectable

KEY POINTS

- Aging of the periocular region includes changes to the periocular skin, orbicularis oculi, ligamentous attachments, and fat.
- Injectable hyaluronic acid (HA) may include a variety of products administered with both cannula and/or needle techniques.
- New study protocols describe more dilute poly-L-lactic acid formulations with combined administration algorithms.
- Periocular platelet-rich plasma (PRP) injections and topical applications are increasingly studied with mixed results.
- Calcium hydroxyapatite administration provides both benefits and detractions when compared with other periocular rejuvenation agents.

INTRODUCTION

Rejuvenation of the periocular region can be a challenging endeavor for any facial plastic surgeon. However, treatment of lower eyelid "bags," a "tired appearance," or "tear trough" deformities are common requests from patients. Increasingly, nonsurgical treatment options are used by both surgeons and nonsurgeons alike to provide a refreshed result. Modern facial plastic surgeons must make the nuanced decision to decide whether surgery is the better option or to use a dermal filler or volumizing agent. This summary aims to provide an updated review of injectable options available to rejuvenate the lower eyelid – cheek junction. Please see other articles in this issue for the treatment of periocular pigmentation and vascularity and use of resurfacing and tightening devices.

ANATOMY

Aging of the lower eyelid–cheek junction is a predictable process that involves the skin, muscle, fat, and ligaments. Each anatomic structure must be considered when rejuvenating this delicate area.[1]

The lower eyelid skin overlying the infraorbital rim continues to thin with time, loses elasticity, suffers sun-related dyschromias, and develops increased laxity and redundancy, or dermatochalasis. Subciliary horizontal rhytids and the more lateral "crow's feet" contribute to an aged appearance. Further, as the epidermal rete ridges decrease in height and number and dermal collagen loses density the skin thins and fails to adequately camouflage the loss of volume along the infraorbital rim.

Attenuation of the orbicularis oculi muscle, divided into the pretarsal, preseptal, and preorbital divisions, leads to decreased lower lid dynamic and static support and further reveals the lid-cheek junction. Also, festoons can form over the malar eminence due to the laxity of the inferior orbicularis oculi muscle draped over the bony orbital rim or edema within the overlying skin.

Ligamentous laxity over time also leads to clear signs of aging (**Fig. 1**). The inferior orbital septum

[a] Ascentist Plastic Surgery, 4801 College Boulevard, Leawood, KS 66211, USA; [b] Dr. Matthew White Facial Plastic Surgery, 800A 5th Ave #502a, New York, NY 10065, USA
* Corresponding author. 6815 E. Frontage Rd, Merriam, KS 66208.
E-mail address: Jeff.markey@ascentist.com

Facial Plast Surg Clin N Am 30 (2022) 321–329
https://doi.org/10.1016/j.fsc.2022.03.006

lies deep to the orbicularis oculi muscle and superficial to the 3 inferior orbital fat pads. The superior margin of the septum is suspended by the tarsus from the medial to lateral canthi, with the inferior border attaching to the orbital rim. With progressive laxity of the orbital septum, the orbital fat pads settle anteriorly, leading to "pseudoherniation" and eye "bags." The orbitomalar ligament is an osteocutaneous ligament originating immediately anterior to the orbital septum along the infraorbital rim extending anteriorly to the skin at the lid-cheek junction. It traverses the orbicularis oculi muscle and lies superior to the SOOF (suborbicularis oculi fat). Nasal to the medial limbus, the orbitomalar ligament attenuates as the orbicularis oculi become tightly adherent to the medial infraorbital rim.

Age-related changes to orbital and superior cheek fat of the lower periocular complex also lead to common patient concerns. The 3 aforementioned lower orbital fat pads are separated by the inferior oblique muscle (medially and centrally) and the arcuate expansion of Lockwood's ligament (centrally and laterally). As the orbital septum becomes laxer with time an unwanted lower lid convexity becomes visible. Further, with the descent and deflation of the SOOF, the infraorbital rim is revealed, forming a "tear trough" deformity. Ligamentous laxity and deflation of the fat lead to the classic double convexity deformity (**Fig. 2**). The superior convexity refers to the aforementioned pseudoherniation of the orbital fat pads. The inferior convexity refers to the settling of the SOOF inferior to the orbitomalar ligament. The convexities are separated by the infraorbital rim.

Understanding the "ideal," youthful anatomy of the lower eyelid–cheek junction is essential, as is understanding the changes associated with aging in the region when considering injectable options in one's practice. A rejuvenated, refreshed lower eyelid and lid–cheek junction involves the anatomic position of the lateral canthus, the tarsus, the orbital fat pads, the orbital septum, the orbitomalar ligament, and the SOOF. The lateral canthus should provide a positive tilt and be positioned 1–2 mm higher than the medial canthus.[2] The tarsus should remain moderately taut against the globe without exposing the inferior limbus to allow for proper lateral-to-medial tear conduction but be elastic enough to allow digital displacement from the infraorbital rim on examination. The orbital septum should support the 3 inferior orbital fat pads to allow a seamless transition from the lash line through the lid–cheek junction. Finally, the orbitomalar ligament and SOOF should be positioned to enable a smooth contour to the

lower eyelid–cheek junction and not expose the infraorbital rim. Injectable fillers can be used to camouflage anatomic changes related to the aging process to restore a youthful appearance.

HYALURONIC ACID

Hyaluronic acid (HA) injectables were first FDA-approved to correct facial contour deformities with the approval of Restylane in 2003. Since this time, the FDA approved additional HA fillers including, chronologically, Juvéderm® (Allergan Pharmaceuticals, Irvine, CA), Belotero® (Merz Aesthetics, Raleigh, NC), RHA® 2, 3, and 4 (Revance Therapeutics, Nashville, TN), among others.[3] The duration of each product's effect and viscosity differ based on the degree of cross-linking, HA concentration, and molecular weight.[4,5] HA fillers are also characterized by a quantitative descriptor G' (G prime). G' refers to the elasticity of the filler, or how well the product retains its shape after a force is applied. Higher G' products are firmer, more easily palpated, and are often placed by injectors in deeper planes to lift tissues. Lower G' products are softer, more easily spread within a tissue plane, and are often placed by injectors in more superficial planes to contour tissues.

Acknowledgment of the wide variability in tear trough correction techniques led to a literature review by Trinh and colleagues[6] The review identified needle injection techniques via aliquots placed in the preperiosteal plane as the most commonly used technique. Restylane was the most commonly used HA product among the reports that met the study criteria.

As the HA product options continue to grow each year, with varying viscosities, durations, and marketing strategies, the injector must strive to stay current to provide the most efficacious results. More specifically, the challenging anatomy of the lower lid–cheek junction forces the modern injector to choose carefully. For example, a high level of cross-linking and larger particle size likely extend product duration but may increase water absorption and subsequent edema.[7] When administering HA products, the ideal endpoint is to slightly underfill the volume deficit to account for their hydrophilic nature.

Juvéderm® Voluma XC (Allergan Pharmaceuticals, Irvine, CA) is a tightly cross-linked, less hygroscopic HA filler that retains contour improvements for up to 2 years.[8] Common usage for higher G' products such as Juvéderm® Voluma XC, RHA 4, Restylane Lyft, among others, involves placement in deeper anatomic planes such as preperiosteal or submuscular to treat anatomic

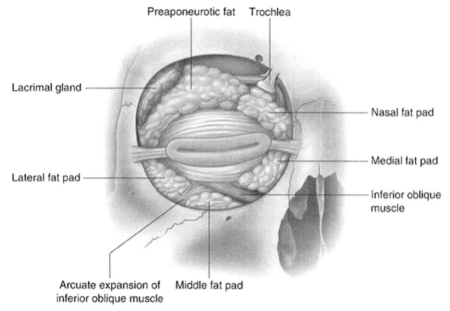

Preaponeurotic fat   Trochlea

Lacrimal gland

Nasal fat pad

Medial fat pad

Inferior oblique
muscle

Lateral fat pad

Arcuate expansion of   Middle fat pad
inferior oblique muscle

Fig. 1. The nasal and middle fat pads are separated anteriorly by the inferior oblique muscle. The lateral fat pad is separated anteriorly from the middle fat pad by the arcuate expansion. (Reprinted by permission from Tan, K.S., Oh, SR., Priel, A., Korn, B.S., Kikkawa, D.O. (2011). Surgical Anatomy of the Forehead, Eyelids, and Midface for the Aesthetic Surgeon. In: Massry, G., Murphy, M., Azizzadeh, B. (eds) Master Techniques in Blepharoplasty and Periorbital Rejuvenation. Springer, New York, NY. https://doi.org/10.1007/978-1-4614-0067-7_2.)

regions such as the malar eminences, temples, chin, and mandibular angles. However, Hall and colleagues reported high rates of patient satisfaction with Juvéderm® Voluma XC administered to the infraorbital hollows.[9] The authors divide the infraorbital hollow into 3 anatomically distinct regions: the medial tear trough, the central nasojugal fold, and the lateral palpebromalar groove. They

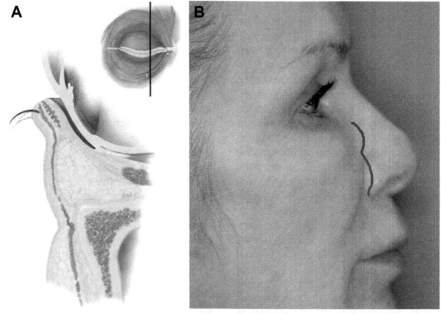

A   B

Fig. 2. (A) Sagittal view of the double convexity deformity. Increased laxity of the orbital septum allows for anterior displacement of the lower orbital fat pads. Descent of the malar fat exposes the infraorbital rim and forms second convexity in the superior cheek. (B) Clinical photo of a double-convexity deformity. ([A] Haddock, Nicholas T. M.D.; Saadeh, Pierre B. M.D.; Boutros, Sean M.D.; Thorne, Charles H. M.D. The Tear Trough and Lid/Cheek Junction: Anatomy and Implications for Surgical Correction, Plastic and Reconstructive Surgery: April 2009 - Volume 123 - Issue 4 - p 1332-1340 doi: 10.1097/PRS.0b013e31819f2b36.; [B] photos courtesy of Dr Jessyka Lighthall.)

placed 0.5 cc of filler on each side using a 27g 1.5-inch Dermasculpt Microcannula® (CosmoFrance Inc., Miami, FL) in the preperiosteal or submuscular planes. Before injection, an infraorbital nerve block was performed via an intraoral approach. Follow-up showed 18 of the 52 patients required touch-up procedures defined as additional filler placed within 3 months of the initial injection. Most patients completing the postprocedure FACE-Q Satisfaction with Eyes Questionnaire reported significant satisfaction with the injections.

Hussain and colleagues reported a needle technique involving Juvéderm® Ultra Plus XC aliquots to the undereye.[10] The authors describe an algorithmic volume predetermination based on Hirman's three grades of tear trough deformity. The authors call this the "tick" method as the 3 anatomic points of filler deposition resemble a checkmark. Zone "A" was located at a point between the inferolateral aspect of the tear trough and the nasojugal groove aligned with the midpupillary line (Fig. 3). Zone "B" was medial, 1–2 cm inferolateral to the medial canthus along the infraorbital rim. Zone "C" is lateral, 1 cm lateral to the lateral limbus at the lid–cheek junction. Subjects with Hirman classes 1, 2, and 3 received 0.3 mL, 0.4 mL, and 0.5 mL, respectively, on each side, spread across the 3 zones as mentioned above. Juvéderm® Ultra Plus XC was backfilled into BD U-40 insulin syringes with 6 mm 31g needles—one for each side. 15% of subjects required additional filler for optimal results at the time of the initial injection. 92% of subjects reported "exceptional improvement" or "very improved" 1 year after the procedure.

Regardless of the specific HA administration technique for the undereye, the injector must understand the risks of HA injection in this region and the most effective management strategies for possible adverse outcomes. These complications can be classified as either acute or long term. Acute complications, including bruising and contour deformities, are normally associated with the injection technique and makeup 90% of the total adverse events.[11] Another acute complication, vascular compromise with or without vision loss, is very rare but a devastating adverse event. Bruising most often occurs secondary to direct vascular injury with either needle or cannula. Avoidance strategies include holding antithrombotic and antiplatelet medications or supplements before injection, applying ice immediately before and after injection, minimizing travel distances of the needle or cannula subdermally, and ensuring injection are placed in an avascular plane such as preperiosteally. Contour deformities include palpable boluses of HA that are inadequately

camouflaged, as well as overfilled tear troughs. Management of filler "nodules" is often treated with firm massage alone, or dispersal with hyaluronidase if persistent. Overfilled tear troughs may appear in the first few days to a few weeks following injection and may be related to the hydrophilic nature of HA fillers. Management of these contour deformities includes watchful waiting for 3 weeks to allow swelling resolution or dispersal with hyaluronidase if persistent.[12] Finally, intravascular injection and downstream occlusion with HA particulate can result in vascular occlusion and periocular soft tissue necrosis. When identified in the acute setting one must set out to restore perfusion by flooding the region with hyaluronidase, applying nitropaste topically, local massage and heat application, and oral administration of aspirin 325 mg.[13] Vision loss may result from retrograde passage of HA filler to occlude the ophthalmic and central retinal arteries. This is treated in the acute setting with the aforementioned treatments as well as supratrochlear and supraorbital hyaluronidase injection, rebreathing into a bag, and ocular massage. A recent consensus statement recommended against retrobulbar hyaluronidase injection.[14,15]

Long-term adverse events include the Tyndall effect and delayed onset nodules. The Tyndall effect occurs when a bluish-gray tint is evident in the tear trough following superficial HA injection. This has been described as occurring anywhere from a few weeks following injection to months or years.[11] To treat the Tyndall effect deformity one may perform dermal treatments to thicken the skin and reduce its transparency, or disperse the filler with hyaluronidase. Delayed onset nodules can occur any time after the acute setting and may follow local trauma to the undereye, filler migration, or infection. When identified, accurately diagnosing the inciting event is essential. If following local trauma, injection with an intralesional steroid such as triamcinolone or 5-fluorouracil may be helpful. If a delayed nodule forms following filler migration dispersal with hyaluronidase should be performed.[13] Finally, if concerned about infection one should treat empirically with broad-spectrum antibiotics including macrolides or tetracyclines following a culture, if possible.

POLY-L-LACTIC ACID

Injectable poly-L-lactic acid (PLLA) (Sculptra®, Galderma, Lausanne, Switzerland) is a biodegradable, immunologically inert, synthetic polymer that provides facial volumization through the stimulation of an inflammatory tissue response with subsequent collagen deposition with dermal

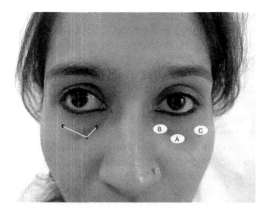

Fig. 3. Patient illustrating "Tick" technique points of injection. (*From*: Hussain SN, Mangal S, Goodman GJ. The Tick technique: A method to simplify and quantify treatment of the tear trough region. J Cosmet Dermatol. 2019 Dec;18(6):1642-1647; reprinted with permission.)

fibroplasia. Sculptra initially received FDA approval for the restoration and correction of HIV-associated facial lipoatrophy in August 2004 and has received approval for broader aesthetic indications.[16]

The distinctive mechanism of action of PLLA compared with other facial fillers provides both benefits and detractions regarding the rejuvenation of the periocular region. HA fillers are largely predictable, lead to an immediate result for real-time feedback, and are able to precisely treat specific facial deficiencies (eg, lines, folds, attenuated lips) with low rates of adverse reactions. In comparison, PLLA is designed to provide volumetric expansion more broadly in volume-deficient areas.[17] PLLA injection leads to delayed results, albeit longer lasting, and usually requires multiple injection sessions spaced 4 to 6 weeks apart for optimal results. PLLA, however, can provide substantial volumization when placed in a supraperiosteal plane and can treat medium to deeply etched lines and wrinkles via collagen deposition when placed in a subcutaneous plane.[10] PLLA boasts an improvement in skin texture and firmness as well.[16]

Various techniques and dilution strategies have been published without consistent protocols among authors. These technical disparities reflect the pursuit of PLLA injectors to minimize the medium and long-term adverse events associated with PLLA administration, without one gold standard approach. The most common complications include contour irregularities or nodules shortly after injection, or delayed granulomatous reactions months to years after injection.[10] Lam and colleagues described injecting 1 to 2 vials per

rejuvenation session when applied to the full face.[17] The authors suggest diluting each vial with 6.5 cc of sterile water and 2 cc of a lidocaine mixture for patient comfort for a total dilution of 8.5 cc for each vial. This additional volume is more diluted than former administration techniques, which often called for as little as 2 cc diluent per vial. The authors also recommended diluting each vial at least 12 hours before injection to allow for more even distribution. Injections to the tear trough area included 0.1 cc preperiosteal depot injections, 0.5 cc on each side in total spread across 5 sites. Circular massage was recommended for each participant for 3 minutes, three times daily, for 3 days. The authors noted the immediate aesthetic changes in facial volume that resulted after the injection of the 8 cc volume of diluted Sculptra approximated the long-term results, with collagen deposition and dermal fibroplasia, after 3 total injection sessions.

Scheirle and Casas performed a similar dilution to study malar augmentation, effacement of the orbitomalar groove, and undereye correction.[16] The authors describe the administration of depot injections, 0.05 cc to 1 cc of product per cm^2 of the surface area to be injected. The injections were placed in the immediate subdermal plane across the malar region and undereye rather than preperiosteally. The authors emphasize the importance of a concurrent topical regimen as well. The study protocol involved the administration of 0.025% tretinoin QHS until tolerated, gradually increasing to 0.05% tretinoin. A portion of the subjects included a hydroquinone-based product to ease distribution and help reduce the incidence of hyperpigmentation. The authors state the beneficial effects of tretinoin—improved skin quality, vascularity, and collagen synthesis—have a synergistic effect with the collagen deposition found with Sculptra Aesthetic. The study reported 99.1% patient satisfaction with a 4.7% incidence of nodule formation at the injection site, with all but one resolving spontaneously.

PLATELET-RICH PLASMA

Platelet-rich plasma (PRP) is also commonly used by facial plastic surgeons to improve skin texture and undereye contours. PRP is a derivative of autologous whole blood with 4 to 7 times the physiologic concentration of platelets. The clinical benefit of PRP injection or topical administration results from activated platelets' release of multiple growth factors, including platelet-derived growth factor, transforming growth factor-B, fibroblast growth factor, epidermal growth factor, keratinocyte growth factor, and vascular endothelium growth factor.[19,20] PRP has been administered both topically and via injection for multiple indications including wound healing, orthopedic indications, dermatologic conditions, and hair restoration.

A review performed by Frautschi and colleagues highlights the multiple current aesthetic uses of PRP, as well as the lack of consistency regarding techniques, preparation processes, and platelet concentration.[21] The authors identified 38 studies meeting the criteria. The studies described injection into aging skin (29%), scalp alopecia (26%), lipofilling (21%), fractional laser uses (13%), and facial surgery (11%). They note that 95% of these studies report clinical benefits to PRP usage. However, only 47% of the studies used objective measures to evaluate these benefits. Despite this lack of consistent efficacy measures the clinical benefit of PRP for aesthetic purposes, including undereye applications, is well described, but further randomized clinical trials or meta-analyses are needed.[22] To better aggregate PRP research moving forward, Frautschi and colleagues recommended a description of the PRP studied to be categorized within the FITPAAW system—centrifugation Force, Iteration (sequence), Time, Platelet concentration, Anticoagulation, Activation, and White Blood Cells. Future reviews may be improved when able to more directly compare PRP harvest, preparation, and administration techniques with objective, quantifiable methods.

Split-face trials serve as some of the best comparisons regarding aesthetic PRP outcomes. Alam and colleagues performed a split-face trial that assessed 19 subjects undergoing mid-dermal PRP serial punctures with a 25g needle spaced 1 cm apart to the cheek and undereye.[23] The contralateral side received saline injections and only one treatment was performed. Both the patient and the dermatologists that served as objective reviewers posttreatment were masked. Photos were taken, and subject self-assessment scores were gathered at 2 weeks, 3 months, and 6 months after the treatment. Two blinded dermatologists reviewed each photo and noted no statistically significant difference regarding fine lines, mottled pigmentation, roughness, and sallowness between halves. However, the subjects' self-assessment scores noted significant improvement regarding pigmentation, texture, wrinkles, and telangiectasias favoring the PRP half. This significant improvement was not detected until the 6-month posttreatment questionnaire and was not noted at 2 weeks or 3 months. The authors' concluded that the improvements may be subtle and thus were not identified by the blinded dermatologists using two-dimensional photography; while the

subjects might have been more easily able to scrutinize differences in the mirror. The study also highlights that a much longer time was needed to appreciate improvements following undereye PRP intradermal injections, as the beneficial changes were delayed until the 6-month questionnaire.

Topical PRP application to the periorbital region performed concurrently with resurfacing or microneedling treatments is also a commonly performed modality. Microneedling uses multiple intradermal, small punctures to facilitate the absorption of topical serums or medications. Even without topical application of PRP, microneedling alone has been shown to increase collagen production, skin tightening, and subjective improvement in skin quality.[24] The microneedling depth and technique are chosen by the practitioner to achieve an endpoint of erythema with or without pinpoint bleeding. PRP can be applied topically during or after microneedling sessions.

Asif and colleagues performed a split-face study to assess the effect of microneedling, with or without PRP, on facial atrophic scarring.[25] The study included 50 subjects. The treatment involved injecting 1 cc of PRP, mixed with 0.1 mL of 10% calcium chloride, with a density of 0.1 mL/cm2. An additional 1 cc of PRP, again mixed with 0.1 mL of 10% calcium chloride, was applied topically. The contralateral side underwent microneedling with intradermal injection of distilled water. A total of 3 sessions were performed at monthly intervals. Using Goodman's Qualitative Scale, the PRP treated side showed a 62.20% improvement compared with 45.84% for the contralateral side, a statistically significant benefit. Both self-reported subject scores and independent dermatologist reviewers further confirmed a statistically significant improvement.

CALCIUM HYDROXYLAPATITE

Lastly, calcium hydroxylapatite (Radiesse®, Merz, Raleigh, NC) is less often used to treat infraorbital volume deficits than other modalities listed in this summary. CaHA was initially FDA approved in 2006 for subdermal administration to correct moderate to severe facial wrinkles such as the nasolabial folds. A review performed by Emer and Sundaram found that CaHA has a good safety profile compared with HA fillers and boasts an immediate volume replacement when applied to the deep dermis in the nasolabial folds which may persist up to 12 months after injection, followed by a longer term deficit improvement secondary to collagenesis.[26] Studies mentioned in the review illustrate the longevity of 30 months or more

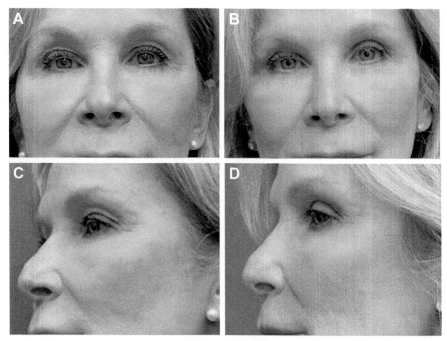

Fig. 4. A/C. Pre and B/D 2-weeks postinjection with calcium hydroxylapatite (Radiesse) in the cheek to treat the double-convexity deformity. (Photos courtesy of Dr Jessyka Lighthall).

regarding nasolabial fold injection. However, CaHA is not fully reversible like HA fillers. The injectable implant is also more viscous than HA fillers and is thus often avoided by facial plastic surgeons in the lid–cheek junction region due to concern for contour deformities.

However, CaHA continues to serve in the armamentarium of facial plastic surgeons seeking to rejuvenate the lid–cheek junction. The viscosity of the product provides substantial lift to ptotic soft tissues such as the superior cheek (Fig. 4). Also, while both HA and CaHA when placed in the tear trough can result in adverse events such as blindness, CaHA may be chosen to reduce complication risk.[27] For these reasons and others CaHA administration to the periorbital complex continues to be an area of active study.

Bernadini and colleagues followed 63 patients undergoing tear trough deformity correction with Radiesse.[28] The technique described involved adding 0.5 cc 2% lidocaine to the 1.5 cc Radiesse vials. Most patients received 1 cc of this mixture in each side. Via a 25g cannula, the product was threaded in a retrograde fashion deep to the orbicularis oculi muscle to achieve the desired effect. As opposed to the slight under correction that is ideal with HA periorbital injections, the authors describe the ideal endpoint as a slight overfill of the volume deficit. The study notes a 92% improvement rate, with 36.5% of patients requiring an additional treatment at 1 month. No patient reported irregular contours, palpable lumpiness, or unevenness. However, 17.4% of patients noted a yellowish discoloration of the skin, which regressed in all cases within 6 weeks. Other nonrandomized case series document similar satisfaction rates with minimal adverse events.[29,30]

SUMMARY

Nonsurgical rejuvenation of the undereye region remains an evolving topic. Each year new volumizing injectables, resurfacing and skin-tightening treatments, and topicals are introduced. The modern facial plastic surgeon must understand the risks, benefits, and alternatives to both the established treatment protocols and the recently developed options.

Hyaluronic acid fillers, poly-L-lactic acid, PRP, and calcium hydroxylapatite are all established rejuvenation options with prior studies documenting reasonable safety profiles. However, each treatment modality varies according to patient expense, risk of adverse events, the longevity of volume deficit improvement, overlying skin changes, and method of administration. It is up to the individual practitioner to identify which products, if any, provide the most efficacious results in their hands.

While there may be a lack of general consensus regarding the ideal technique or product, practitioners can agree that the rejuvenation of the lower lid–cheek junction is a challenging procedure with a steep learning curve and serious complication risk. Before attempting the rejuvenation of this area, injectors should have intimate knowledge of the periorbital anatomy, practical experience with various injection techniques, and an understanding of how to manage complications should they arise.

CLINICS CARE POINTS

- Choosing specific non-surgical modalities to rejuvenate the periocular complex requires in-depth knowledge of the delicate anatomy.
- Each modality - HA, PLLA, PRP, CaHa - has various advantages and disadvantages and should be used with distinct clinical endpoints in mind.

DISCLOSURE

The authors report no commercial or financial conflicts of interest and report no funding sources for this article.

REFERENCES

1. Alghoul M, Codner MA. Retaining ligaments of the face: review of anatomy and clinical applications. Aesthet Surg J 2013;33(6):769–82.
2. Tepper OM, Steinbrech D, Howell MH, et al. A retrospective review of patients undergoing lateral canthoplasty techniques to manage existing or potential lower eyelid malposition: identification of seven key preoperative findings. Plast Reconstr Surg 2015;136:40–9.
3. FDA. Executive Summary general issues Panel meeting on dermal fillers prepared for the meeting of the general and plastic surgery devices Advisory Panel. Available at: https://www.fda.gov/media/146870/download.
4. Lee S, Yen M. Nonsurgical Rejuvenation of the Eyelids with Hyaluronic Acid Gel Injections. Semin Plast Surg 2017;31(01):017–21.
5. Anido J, et al. Recommendations for the treatment of tear trough deformity with crosslinked hyaluronic acid filler. J Cosmet Dermatol 2021;20:6–17.
6. Trinh LN, Grond SE. Amar Gupta, Dermal Fillers for Tear Trough Rejuvenation: A Systematic Review.

Facial Plast Surg 2021. https://doi.org/10.1055/s-0041-1731348.
7. Anido J, Fernández JM, Genol I, et al. Recommendations for the treatment of tear trough deformity with crosslinked hyaluronic acid filler. J Cosmet Dermatol 2021;20(1):6–17.
8. Few J, Cox SE, Paradkar-Mitragotri D, et al. A Multicenter, Single-Blind Randomized, Controlled Study of a Volumizing Hyaluronic Acid Filler for Midface Volume Deficit: Patient-Reported Outcomes at 2 Years. Aesthet Surg J 2015;35(5):589–99.
9. Hall MB, Roy S, Buckingham ED. Novel Use of a Volumizing Hyaluronic Acid Filler for Treatment of Infraorbital Hollows. JAMA Facial Plast Surg 2018;20(5):367–72.
10. Hussain SN, Mangal S, Goodman GJ. The Tick technique: A method to simplify and quantify treatment of the tear trough region. J Cosmet Dermatol 2019;18(6):1642–7.
11. Murthy R, Roos JCP, Goldberg RA. Periocular hyaluronic acid fillers. Curr Opin Ophthalmol 2019;30(5):395–400.
12. DeLorenzi C. Complications of injectable fillers, part 1. Aesthet Surg J 2013;33:561–75.
13. Jordan DR, Stoica B. Filler migration: a number of mechanisms to consider. Ophthal Plast Reconstr Surg 2015;31:257–62.
14. Beer K, Downie J, Beer J. A treatment protocol for vascular occlusion from particulate soft tissue augmentation. J Clin Aesthet Dermatol 2012;5(5):44–7.
15. Humzah DM, Ataullah S, Chiang C, et al. The treatment of hyaluronic acid aesthetic interventional induced visual loss (AIIVL): a consensus on practical guidance. J Cosmet Dermatol 2019;18:71–6.
16. Schierle CF, Casas LA. Nonsurgical Rejuvenation of the Aging Face With Injectable Poly-L-Lactic Acid for Restoration of Soft Tissue Volume. Aesthet Surg J 2011;31(1):95–109.
17. Lam SM, Azizzadeh B, Graivier M. Injectable Poly-L-Lactic Acid (Sculptra): Technical Considerations in Soft-Tissue Contouring. Plast Reconstr Surg 2006;118(Suppl):55S–63S.
18. Sadick NS, Manhas-Bhutani S, Krueger N. A Novel Approach to Structural Facial Volume Replacement. Aesthet Plast Surg 2013;37(2):266–76.
19. Alves R, Grimalt R. A review of platelet-rich plasma: history, biology, mechanism of action, and classification. Skin Appendage Disord 2018;4(1):18–24.
20. Peng GL. Platelet-Rich Plasma for Skin Rejuvenation: Facts, Fiction, and Pearls for Practice. Facial Plast Surg Clin North Am 2019;27(3):405–11.
21. Frautschi RS, Hashem AM, Halasa B, et al. Current evidence for clinical efficacy of platelet rich plasma in aesthetic surgery: a systematic review. Aesthet Surg J 2017;37(3):353–62.

22. Evans AG, Ivanic MG, Botros MA, et al. Rejuvenating the periorbital area using platelet-rich plasma: a systematic review and meta-analysis. Arch Dermatol Res 2021;313:711–27.

23. Alam M, Hughart R, Champlain A, et al. Effect of Platelet-Rich Plasma Injection for Rejuvenation of Photoaged Facial Skin: A Randomized Clinical Trial. JAMA Dermatol 2018;154(12):1447–52.

24. Chamata Edward SMD, Bartlett Erica LMD, Weir David NP-C, et al. Platelet-Rich Plasma: Evolving Role in Plastic Surgery. Plast Reconstr Surg January 2021;147(1):219–30.

25. Asif M, Kanodia S, Singh K. Combined autologous platelet-rich plasma with microneedling verses microneedling with distilled water in the treatment of atrophic acne scars: a concurrent split-face study. J Cosmet Dermatol 2016;15(4):434–43.

26. Emer J, Sundaram H. Aesthetic applications of calcium hydroxylapatite volumizing filler: an evidence-based review and discussion of current concepts: (part 1 of 2). J Drugs Dermatol 2013;12(12): 1345–54.

27. Chatrath V, Banerjee PS, Goodman GJ, et al. Soft-tissue Filler-associated Blindness: A Systematic Review of Case Reports and Case Series. Plast Reconstr Surg Glob Open 2019;7(4):e2173.

28. Bernardini FP, Cetinkaya A, Devoto MH, et al. Calcium hydroxyl-apatite (Radiesse) for the correction of periorbital hollows, dark circles, and lower eyelid bags. Ophthal Plast Reconstr Surg 2014;30(1):34–9.

29. Wollina U, Goldman A. Long lasting facial rejuvenation by repeated placement of calcium hydroxylapatite in elderly women. Dermatol Ther 2020;33(6): e14183.

30. Jacovella PF. Use of calcium hydroxylapatite (Radiesse) for facial augmentation. Clin Interv Aging 2008;3(1):161–74.

Carbon Dioxide Laser Rejuvenation of the Facial Skin

Kasra Ziai, MD[a], Harry V. Wright, MD, MS[b],*

KEYWORDS

• Laser • Carbon dioxide laser • Facial rejuvenation • Facial resurfacing

KEY POINTS

• It is imperative to identify the goals of the patient and his or her definition of an optimal outcome.
• A careful patient examination and a solid foundational understanding of basic laser physics are important to determine if the proposed intervention can meet those goals.
• Facial skin resurfacing is focused on reestablishing the smooth, elastic, and firm appearance characteristic of youthful skin.
• Advances in both technology, techniques, and pre and postoperative skincare allow for significant skin tightening, reduction in rhytid burden, high patient satisfaction, and a manageable side effect/complication profile.

INTRODUCTION

Aesthetic rejuvenation of the facial skin focuses on restoring the quality and contour of the skin with special attention to a regional harmony of the final outcome. As individuals age, the skin of the face and neck thins, loses elasticity, and develops dyspigmentations, textural irregularities, and rhytids as photoaging accumulates. Under the combined influences of gravity, the mimetic musculature of the face, soft tissue volume alterations, and physical habits (such as unfavorable sleep positioning or tobacco use) both fine and coarse creases develop. These changes characterize the individuals' dissatisfaction with the appearance of their facial skin and their desire to seek correction.

Various surgical and nonsurgical techniques are used alone or in combination to restore a youthful appearance to the facial skin and deliver the desired result of restoration. Laser resurfacing offers the advantage of improved control and reproducibility in comparison to traditional methods of chemical peeling and dermabrasion, though these are still used in aesthetic facial rejuvenation.[1,2] Although other types of therapy exist to target the components of photoaging (eg, erbium:yag, Nd:YAG, IPL, PDL, and so forth), one of the most commonly used treatments for resurfacing is the CO_2 laser. CO_2 lasers induce a thermal wound which provides the characteristic ability to both coagulate and induce intense collagen remodeling within the dermis.[3–5]

In this article, we focus on the fractionated CO_2 laser, long considered the gold standard for facial skin rejuvenation. Although many different devices exist, what follows is a description of how the senior author uses an Ultrapulse CO2 laser (Ultra-Pulse Encore; Lumenis Ltd, Yokneam, Israel), customizing the procedure to each patient with the principles and rationale behind each protocol.

Funding/Support: None.

[a] Department of Otolaryngology–Head and Neck Surgery, The Pennsylvania State University, Milton S. Hershey Medical Center, Hershey, PA 17033, USA; [b] Wright Spellman Plastic Surgery, 5911 N. Honore Avenue, Suite 120, Sarasota, FL 34243, USA
* Corresponding author. Wright Spellman Plastic Surgery, 5911 N. Honore Avenue, Suite 120, Sarasota, FL 34243.
E-mail address: dr.hvwright@gmail.com

Facial Plast Surg Clin N Am 30 (2022) 331–346
https://doi.org/10.1016/j.fsc.2022.03.007

BASIC LASER PHYSICS

Lasers emit light energy that travels in a waveform, as does ordinary light. The wavelength is the distance between 2 successive peaks of a wave (Fig. 1). The amplitude is the height of the peak and is related to the intensity of the light. Frequency (or period) is the amount of time required for one full wave cycle.[6,7]

To understand laser function it is important for the operator to understand basic laser mechanics. If a photon—the unit of light energy—strikes an atom it boosts one of its electrons to a higher energy level. The "excited" atom is unstable and will reemit a photon as the electron drops to its original lower energy level, a process known as *spontaneous emission*. If that "excited" atom is struck by yet another photon, it will emit 2 photons that have the same wavelength, direction, and phase when the electrons revert to lower energy levels. One can see how a chain reaction may proceed from successive collisions, generating large volumes of coherent light. This process is known as *the stimulated emission* of radiation and is the underlying principle of laser physics.[8–10]

As a laser beam impacts tissue its energy may be absorbed, reflected, transmitted, or scattered, and in laser skin rejuvenation absorption is most important. The extent of absorption depends on the chromophore content of the tissue. Chromophores are substances that absorb the energy of a particular light wavelength efficiently. For example, CO_2 laser energy is absorbed by soft tissues of the body because the target chromophore is water, which makes up 80% of soft tissue content. In contrast, the CO_2 laser has relatively minimal effect on bone (which has a low water content). Initially, as a tissue absorbs the laser energy, its molecules begin to vibrate. Absorption of additional energy causes protein denaturation, coagulation, and, finally, vaporization/ablation.[13,14]

As noted above, the modifiable factor affecting laser-tissue interaction is energy density. Energy density is equal to the power density of the incident beam multiplied by the exposure time. Power density is the power expressed in watts divided by the cross-sectional area of the laser beam (spot size), as in the following equation:

$$Power\ density = \frac{Power(W)}{Cross - sectional\ area\ of\ laser\ beam(spot\ size)}$$

This laser energy is then "collimated"—made dense and parallel—by a system of opposing mirrors within the resonating chamber and then transmitted to the intended target by a delivery system (Fig. 2). Thus, laser light is organized, intense, and diverges very little as it travels, giving laser energy its characteristic constant intensity even over long distances.[10,11]

LASER-TISSUE INTERACTION

A laser can exert a spectrum of effects on biologic tissue, from the modulation of biologic function to vaporization, with the majority of clinically relevant systems using laser's thermal effects to coagulate and/or vaporize tissue.[8,12]

The effect of a particular laser on a specific tissue depends on the following 3 factors: tissue absorption, laser wavelength, and laser energy density.[6,12] The first 2 factors are constant and inherent to the tissue and laser, respectively. Importantly the third factor, energy density, can be manipulated by the surgeon. It is critical that the operator has at least a basic understanding of laser-tissue interaction to provide maximal benefit to the patient and minimize risks.

Power density may be seen as the amount of power (in watts) delivered to the area by the laser. Energy density, also known as fluence, simply adds the dimension of time and is expressed in $joules/cm^2$:

Energy density = power density × time

Therefore, varying the spot size or the exposure time can alter the laser-tissue interaction effects (if all other factors are constant). As the spot size of a laser beam decreases (thereby increasing the power density) the amount of power reaching that particular volume of tissue increases. Conversely, as the spot size increases, the energy density of a laser beam decreases.[15–18]

Pulsing the laser energy is another method by which the surgeon can modify tissue effects via alternating periods of "power on" with periods of "power off." Because energy is not reaching tissue during the off periods, heat is allowed to dissipate during those intervals. If the off periods are longer than the thermal relaxation time of the targeted tissue, there is less risk of damaging the surrounding tissue by the conduction of heat. Energy can be pulsed by setting the time that the laser is on (for

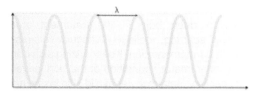

Fig. 1. Laser sine wave pattern. The wavelength (λ) is the distance between two successive peaks of a wave. (*From* Franck P, Henderson PW, Rothaus KO. Basics of Lasers: History, Physics, and Clinical Applications. *Clinics in plastic surgery.* 2016;43(3):505-513.)

example, 0.1 seconds). The energy can be shuttered, where the continuous wave is blocked during specified intervals by a mechanical shutter. In a superpulse mode, the energy is not simply blocked but is stored within the power supply of the laser during the off interval and then released during the on interval. Thus, the peak energy of the superpulse mode greatly exceeds that of the continuous or shuttered modes.[11,19–22]

TREATMENT CONCEPTS

Patients who may benefit from laser skin resurfacing include those with facial rhytids, textural irregularities, photoaging (including seborrheic and actinic keratosis, actinic cheilitis, and dyschromia), and scarring resulting from trauma, iatrogenic causes, or acne.[18,23,24] Patients who are predisposed to cancerous lesions of the face may benefit from prophylactic ablation of subclinical precancerous lesions (personal observation). Facial subunits or the entire face can be treated in one setting, and treatment can be performed concurrently with various other rejuvenation procedures including blepharoplasty and facelift.

Baker has developed a classification system that stratifies the aging process in the soft tissues of the neck and lower face (**Table 1**).[25] The Glogau scale[26] is a useful grading system for the classification of photoaging (**Table 2**) and the Fitzpatrick scale[27] is used to classify skin type and the patient's ethnicity that can determine the safety and effectiveness of resurfacing procedures (**Table 3**).

These classification systems are useful in treatment planning for facial rejuvenation and help develop the safest CO_2 laser protocol allowing for optimal skin resurfacing for each patient. For example, patients with a higher Fitzpatrick level have may be contraindicated for CO_2 resurfacing or have a higher risk of posttreatment dyspigmentation and scarring, and those with an advanced Glogau level may require more aggressive laser resurfacing or serial treatments in combination with other interventions to optimize rejuvenation. As aging is multifaceted, a multimodal treatment plan is often recommended and may include chemodenervation, skin resurfacing, liposuction/lipolysis, volumizing procedures, tightening, and so forth. It is important to identify the particular anatomic target(s) for correction as well as the patient's goals of treatment to determine the best course of rejuvenation and set realistic expectations.

Deep skin resurfacing is indicated for moderate to severe skin laxity characteristic of loss of elasticity, fine rhytidosis, and photoaging. Ideal candidates demonstrate appropriate skin type and skin condition, absence of contraindications, and (importantly) patient acceptance of procedure-specific risks and expected recovery.[28–31] The senior author prefers to treat Fitzpatrick skin types I–II but will treat type III (albeit less aggressively).

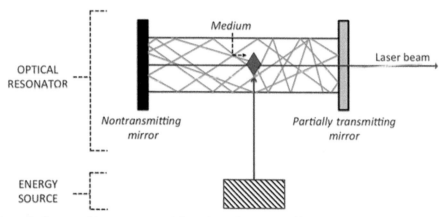

Fig. 2. Schematic diagram of laser component. Laser beam is generated by energy source, activating electrons of medium and subsequent release of protons. The Protons are then reflected by nontransmitting mirror and laser beam is released from partially transmitting mirror. (*From* Franck P, Henderson PW, Rothaus KO. Basics of Lasers: History, Physics, and Clinical Applications. Clinics in plastic surgery. 2016;43(3):505--513.)

Table 1
Baker's classification of the aging process in the soft tissues of the neck and face

Baker's Classification	
Type 1	Slight cervical skin laxity with submental fat and early jowls
Type 2	Moderate cervical skin laxity, moderate jowls, and submental fat
Type 3	Moderate cervical skin laxity, but with significant jowling and active platysmal banding
Type 4	Loose redundant cervical skin and folds below the cricoid, significant jowls, and active platysmal bands

Importantly, patients must be willing to accept up to 2 weeks of downtime during the period of reepithelialization and accept the risks inherent to deep skin resurfacing. These include delayed healing, scarring, prolonged erythema, milia formation, and persistent dyschromia (hyper- and hypo-pigmentation).

Absolute contraindications include active skin infection or other inflammatory or neoplastic cutaneous disease, isotretinoin use within the past year, immunosuppression, melasma, pregnancy, lactation, history of keloids or severe herpes infections, the likelihood of poor compliance, patient nonacceptance regarding postop recovery and downtime, and unrealistic expectations regarding treatment benefits and outcomes.[32,33]

Relative contraindications include prior radiation therapy or deep burn in the treatment area, abnormal scarring, collagen vascular disease, diffuse hyperpigmentation, Koebnerizing skin conditions, inflammatory condition of the skin, severe skin sensitivity, severe lower eyelid skin laxity, and prior lower eyelid surgery.[30]

PRETREATMENT CONSIDERATIONS

Although there is no consensus for an exact protocol, in our practice we prefer to treat patients beginning the night before the resurfacing procedure with oral cephalexin (500 mg BID for 5 days), valacyclovir, and fluconazole to decrease the potential risk of postprocedural bacterial, herpetic, and fungal infections.[34–36] Although prophylactic antibiotic and antifungal therapy remain controversial.[37,38] Patients who are Fitzpatrick skin type III or are prone to postinflammatory hyperpigmentation are treated for 5 weeks prior to the procedure with a topical cream containing 0.1% tretinoin, 5% hydroquinone, and 0.5% hydrocortisone.[39–41]

Patients should arrange for a driver to and from the procedure if anxiolytics, monitored or general anesthesia, or periocular resurfacing are being used.

TREATMENT: SKIN PREPARATION

Treatment should be performed in a well-ventilated room with adequate lighting. In the operating room, CO_2 laser skin resurfacing may be performed concurrently with various other surgical procedures. In either case, the skin should be prepared gently with an appropriate antimicrobial solution per manufacturer protocol. Inflammable alcohol-containing antiseptic solutions should be

Table 2
Glogau photoaging scale

Group	Classification	Age	Characteristics
Group 1 (no wrinkles)	Mild	28–35	Mild pigmentary changes, No keratosis, Minimal or no makeup
Group 2 (wrinkles in motion)	Moderate	35–50	Early senile lentigo, early keratoses, early wrinkles, and parallel smile lines, wears some makeup
Group 3 (wrinkles at rest)	Advanced	50–65	Noticeable dyschromia, telangiectasia, deep wrinkles, visible keratosis always wear makeup
Group 4 (all wrinkles)	Severe	>60	Yellow-grey discoloration, extensive wrinkles, actinic keratosis ± history of skin malignancy, makeup cakes

Table 3
Fitzpatrick sun-reactive skin types

Skin Types	Skin Color	Tanning Response
I	Pale white	Always burns, never tans
II	White	Usually burns, tans with difficulty
III	Light brown	Sometimes burns, usually tans
IV	Moderate brown	Rarely burns, tans very easily
V	Dark brown	Very rarely burns, tans very easily
VI	Deeply dark brown/black	No burn, tans very easily

Skin types I and II are ideal candidates for CO2 laser skin resurfacing. Type III can be treated with CO2 laser but less aggressively.

avoided. The skin surface should be dry at the time of treatment.

TREATMENT: ANESTHESIA

One of the major challenges associated with laser resurfacing procedures is pain. CO_2 laser skin resurfacing can cause considerable discomfort/pain in comparison to other resurfacing procedures related to the deeper penetration and significant stimulation of dermal nerve fibers. This can be alleviated by using local or general anesthesia. Monitored anesthesia care (MAC) and general anesthesia are reserved for patients that appropriate anesthesia cannot be achieved by local anesthetics or in case of concurrent treatment with surgical procedures such as rhytidectomy.

There are multiple types of topical anesthetic agents available. One of the most commonly used topical anesthetic preparations is a Lidocaine 2.5% and Prilocaine 2.5% mixture, also known as EMLA (Astra Pharmaceuticals, Westborough, MA). Occlusion and a prolonged application will increase the penetration of EMLA cream. In most cases, the application of EMLA cream 1 to 2 hours before facial resurfacing can provide appropriate analgesia for most patients.[42,43] Topical anesthesia preparations can impact skin tissue impedance and can unpredictably affect laser-tissue interaction. This concern is related to the hydrophilic nature of topical anesthesia such as EMLA and water is the main chromophore for the CO_2 laser. However, in a study by Naouri and colleagues[44] authors did not find variability in the skin's response to CO_2 fractional resurfacing with the use of local anesthetic using high-resolution ultrasound imaging. This topic remains controversial. LMX4, LMX5, Topicaine®, Lidoderm®, and a mixture of Lidocaine 7% and Tetracaine 7% are among other commonly used topical preparations used for anesthesia.

It is not uncommon that patients will require additional anesthesia with nerve blocks (supraorbital, infraorbital, mental) or tumescent anesthesia that can be infiltrated in the lateral aspects of the face particularly in full-face CO2 laser resurfacing. Preprocedural anxiolytics (given 30 minutes before the procedure) can be helpful in patient comfort and reduce the total amount of local anesthetics necessary to maintain comfort. In a study on 200 patients undergoing CO_2 laser facial resurfacing, a combination of EMLA cream, oral diazepam (5–10 mg), and intramuscular ketorolac (30–60 mg) was demonstrated to provide adequate anesthesia in 95% of cases.[42]

Cold air cooling (cryoanesthesia) is another method to increase patients' comfort while performing laser resurfacing as well as the added benefit of thermal protection.[45,46] Cold air cooling can be used in combination with other local anesthesia methods to provide longer lasting anesthesia.

TREATMENT: SAFETY CONCERNS

The main safety concern in any laser procedure is thermal injury and the potential risk of fire. This is an environmental safety concern with a high risk in CO2 laser procedures that can happen with fractionated oxygen levels above room air (>21%).[47,48] It is recommended to avoid supplemental oxygen (if possible) during the laser procedure. If the procedure is performed under general anesthesia and intubation is required, a laser-safe endotracheal tube should be used. Although most reported CO_2 laser-induced fires are related to oropharyngeal surgery. Cutaneous laser resurfacing seems to be safe. That being said, current recommendations suggest using a laser-safe endotracheal tube or wrapping the endotracheal tube with wet gauze. Additionally, a misfired laser beam can result in igniting patients', physicians', or assistants' clothing.[49] This risk can be mitigated by placing moist towels around the patient's head and neck during the procedure. Labeling the laser foot pedal, availability of fire extinguishers in the procedure room, having an assistant responsible for placing the laser in standby mode when not in use, and having warning signs at the entrance of the procedure room are other factors that can decrease the risk of thermal injury and fire.

Eye protection is required for both patient and physician/personnel. Metal eye/corneal shields should be used for all patients during the procedure to prevent injury to the cornea and retina. Topical ophthalmic drops are used to anesthetize the eyes then lubricating ophthalmic ointment is placed on the shields before insertion. Plastic eye shields are susceptible to thermal damage and should be avoided.[47,50] All procedure/operating room personnel should wear protective goggles with side shields to prevent direct or indirect (reflected from metallic surfaces) damage from the laser beam.

TREATMENT: DEVICE SETTINGS AND ENERGY DELIVERY

The Lumenis Ultrapulse Encore CO_2 laser offers 2 different delivery handpieces/scanners (Active FX and Deep FX) that are used individually or combined, based on the goals and the type of treatment necessary. The Active FX (or CPG) handpiece has a 1.3 mm spot size and delivers the laser beam energy in a nonsequential pattern that minimizes the risk of thermal damage. The Active FX handpiece is used for superficial ablation (fine rhytids, dyschromia, acne scarring) and usually penetrates up to the level of the superficial papillary dermis. It provides 7 different patterns (settings) with different size and density options and delivers energy from 2 mJ (150 mJ/cm2) to 225 mJ (169 J/cm2) and power ranging from 4.4 Hz to 600 Hz. Density settings can range from 1 to 9. Density 1 corresponds to 55% surface ablation while density 4 or greater corresponds to 100% surface ablation (density 2 and 3 correspond to 68% and 82%, respectively). The usual setting for facial resurfacing is 100 to 125 mJ and a density of 2 to 4. These settings should be adjusted for areas with thinner skin such as the periorbital and neck region (energy: 60–90 mJ, density: 1–3).[51,52]

The Deep FX handpiece is used for deep rhytids and scars to enhance collagen regeneration. The spot size for Deep FX (0.12 mm) is significantly narrower than Active FX and penetrates to deep dermis layers. It has four different patterns and six different size options. The settings for the energy range from 2.5 mJ to 50 mJ with the option for one pulse or two-stacked pulses. The usual energy setting for the face is 15 to 22.5 mJ with a density of 5% to 25%. Like Active FX, the settings should be adjusted for the periorbital and neck region (energy: 8–10 mJ, density 5%–15%). If combined with Active FX, then resurfacing with Deep FX should be performed first, followed by superficial resurfacing.

Facial skin resurfacing is focused on reestablishing the smooth, elastic, and firm appearance characteristic of youthful skin. The operator's technique and experience play an important role in achieving optimal results. During the procedure, the foot pedal should be placed in a comfortable position for the operator and the scanner should be held perpendicular to the target area. Immediate edema and pinpoint oozing can occur during CO_2 laser resurfacing that can be cleaned with sterile gauze soaked in saline.

TREATMENT ENDPOINT

The immediate endpoint in superficial CO_2 laser resurfacing (with or without deep resurfacing) is the removal of the epidermal layer of the skin and exposure of the papillary dermis that clinically is distinguishable with yellowing of the wound bed and pinpoint bleeding. If the depth of ablation does not extend beyond the epidermis into the papillary dermis then the likelihood of dramatic results is low, while deeper penetration of high energy laser beam beyond the papillary dermis carries the risk of scaring.

POSTTREATMENT WOUND CARE

During the initial healing period the treated skin must be kept moist with an occlusive dressing or ointment. The desiccated outer skin layers slough in approximately 4 to 10 days as the newly regenerated epithelium appears. Focal areas of slower healing apparent beyond postop day 10 may be spot treated with the same occlusive ointment. Antivirals, topical antifungals, and antibiotics may be continued. Postprocedural skin regimens vary greatly and there is no consensus as to a standard regimen. Following reepithelialization, the ointment is discontinued and both a light moisturizer and extracellular matrix modulators are started. Sun exposure and harsh wind conditions should be avoided for 6 weeks or more following epithelialization. Mineral-based camouflage makeup may be started within a week after reepithelialization, and nonirritating sunscreen may be applied as soon as 3 to 4 weeks.

CO_2 LASER SKIN RESURFACING AS A CONCURRENT TREATMENT

Historically, the combination of skin resurfacing (specifically chemical peels) and rhytidectomy has been a point of controversy and concern. The likelihood of damage to the already compromised blood supply of the raised skin flaps and subsequent skin flap necrosis resulted in recommendations against concurrent treatment. The increased time of recovery after rhytidectomy with full ablative resurfacing procedures was another contributable factor to advise against the combination of these procedures.[53–55]

Recent advances in laser technology including fractionated laser resurfacing and multiple studies demonstrating a low risk of complications with simultaneous therapy have shifted modern medicine to attest to the safety of concurrent CO_2 laser resurfacing with other aging face procedures (rhytidectomy, browlift, blepharoplasty).[56–58] In a meta-analysis of nine studies including 453 patients who underwent concurrent rhytidectomy and laser resurfacing, the reported rate of anterior skin flap necrosis was found to be less than 0.2% (only in one patient).[59]

In concurrent treatment, the usual laser settings for both Deep FX and Active FX are used except over the skin flaps. For Deep FX, the energy of 17.5 to 20 mJ with a power of 350 Hz and density of 15 is recommended. This is followed by Active FX resurfacing (energy: 80–135 mJ, power: 350 Hz, density: 3). However, when performing Active FX resurfacing over the skin flaps and neck the energy and density should be brought down to 60 to 70 mJ and a density of 2.[57]

AVOIDANCE AND MANAGEMENT OF COMPLICATIONS

All facial resurfacing procedures are associated with a risk of postoperative complications that are the result of damage to the skin surface and subsequent launch of the regeneration process. The fractional lasers induce less damage to the skin surface compared with ablative lasers and as a result, the complication rates are lower and less severe when the fractional laser is used for resurfacing procedures.[60]

Postinflammatory hyperpigmentation (PIH) is a common complication of laser resurfacing that usually occurs within the first 3 to 4-weeks posttreatment. It is more common in patients with Fitzpatrick III and higher. In a study of 961 laser resurfacing treatments, the rate of PIH was 33% among patients with Fitzpatrick V skin complexity in comparison to 2.5% in patients with Fitzpatrick

III skin prototype.[60] The incidence of PIH can be minimized by pretreatment (3–8 weeks) of high-risk patients (Fitzpatrick 3 or higher) with retinoic acid, hydroquinone 4%, and hydrocortisone.[61] Treatment is by continuing the same regimen (if tolerated) for 2 to 3-weeks postprocedure.

Infections are another potential complication after skin laser resurfacing. Herpes simplex (HSV) eruptions (1.77%) are more common than fungal and bacterial infections after laser resurfacing. As mentioned before, all patients are started on valacyclovir, fluconazole, and cephalexin 1 day before their treatment in the senior author's practice but these treatments are controversial. If eruptions of herpes vesicles occur, 500 mg to 1 g of valacyclovir should be given daily until reepithelialization is completed (day 10).[62] Posttreatment bacterial infections are most commonly caused by staphylococcus aureus and treatment with 5 to 7 days of cephalexin is recommended. The most common cause of posttreatment fungal infection is candida which is treated with fluconazole (200 mg the first day, and then 100 mg daily for 1–2 weeks). Other regimens may include topical antifungals or antibiotic creams.

Contact dermatitis is another complication that can occur and is typically caused by the use of moisturizer, antibiotic ointment, or makeup. If mild to moderate, then a strong steroid cream is recommended, and if severe, systematic oral steroids should be used.[63,64] Synechia, hypopigmentation, hypertrophic scarring, scleral show (mostly in patients with a history of blepharoplasty), ectropion, and laser injury to the globe are among other potential complications.

CASE STUDIES

The following are the case descriptions performed by a senior author.

PERIORAL CO_2

Case 1 (**Fig. 3**): A case of perioral CO_2 laser skin resurfacing in a 68-year-old female. Pre and postprocedure photos were taken 1 year apart. The Luxar Novapulse CO_2 laser was used to resurface the perioral region in a painting pattern with 25% overlap. The first pass was performed in the E8 mode at 6 W. A second pass was made under the same settings and the papillary dermis was identified. A third pass was made in the E8 mode at 4 W. The final pass was taken over the vermilion border to allow for resurfacing of the vermilion mucosa. Eschar was removed between passes with saline-soaked gauze.

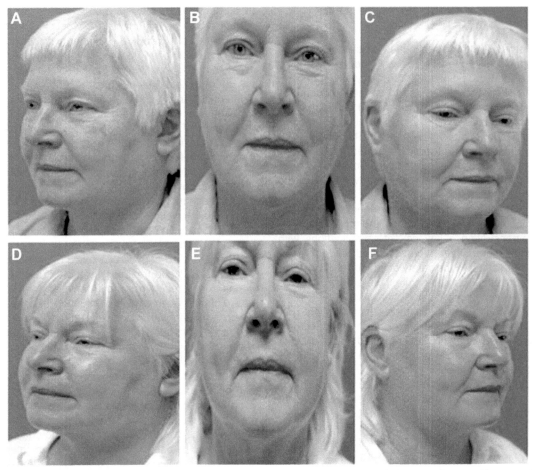

Fig. 3. Preprocedure photos of a 68-year-old female (*A–C*). One-year postperioral Skin resurfacing with Lumenis Ultrapulse CO_2 (*D–F*).

Case 2 (**Fig. 4**): Another case of perioral CO_2 laser skin resurfacing in a 63-year-old female that shows significant improvement of perioral fine rhytids. The Luxar Novapulse CO_2 laser was used to resurface the perioral region in a painting pattern with 25% overlap. The first pass was performed in the E8 mode at 6 W. A second pass was made under the same settings and a papillary dermis was identified. A third pass over the lips whereby the perioral rhytids were most concentrated was made in the E8 mode at 4 W. That final pass was taken over the vermilion border to allow for resurfacing of the vermilion mucosa. Eschar was removed between passes with saline-soaked gauze. Postprocedural photos were taken 1 year after the laser resurfacing.

FULL-FACE CO_2

Case 4 (**Fig. 5**): This case represents concurrent treatment with full-face CO_2 laser resurfacing and facelift in a 62-year-old female. The Lumenis Ultrapulse CO_2 laser was used. The Deep FX handpiece was used to treat the perioral face at the following settings: 25 mJ, density 5%. The remainder of the face (except those areas within the bony orbit) was treated at the following settings: 10 mJ, density 5%. Then, the Active FX handpiece was affixed to the device and the first pass was performed on the lower eyelids and skin contained within the orbital rims (excluding the hair-bearing brow) at the following settings: 80 mJ, 45W, density 4, pattern 5, size 6. A second pass was made. The remaining facial skin (excluding the skin flaps) was treated at the following settings: 100 mJ, 60W, density 1, pattern 1, size 9. The second pass was made in a direction orthogonal to the first, in a similar painting pattern. The facelift skin flaps were then treated with a single pass at 80 mJ, 45W, density 4, pattern 5, size 6. Blending/feathering of the treatment area was performed along the jawline with the handpiece held tangentially to the skin: 80 mJ, 45W, density 3, pattern 1, size 9. The postoperative photo was

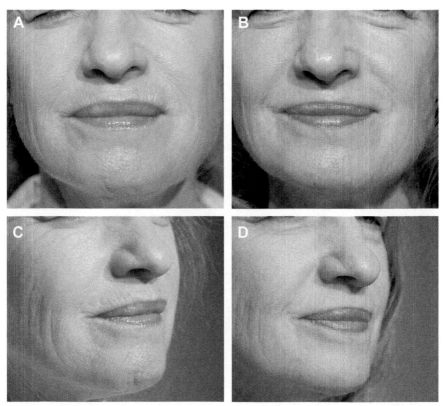

Fig. 4. Photos of a 63-year-old female with perioral fine rhytids (*A, C*). One-year postperioral Skin resurfacing with Lumenis Ultrapulse CO_2 (*B, D*).

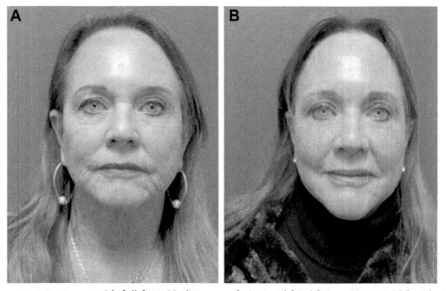

Fig. 5. Concurrent treatment with full-face CO_2 laser resurfacing and facelift in a 62-year-old female. Preoperative photo (*A*). Six-weeks postoperative photo (*B*).

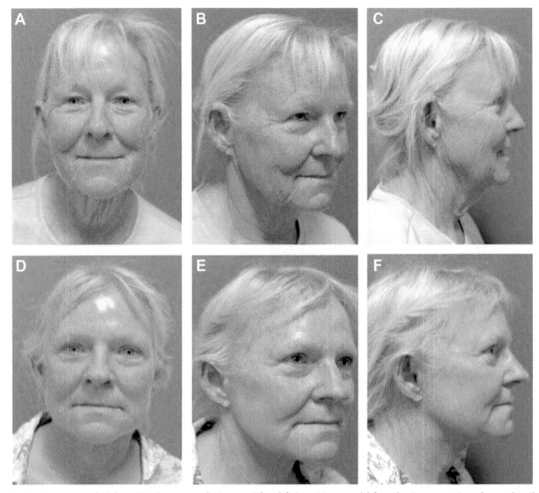

Fig. 6. Concurrent full-face CO_2 laser resurfacing and facelift in a 59-year-old female. Preoperative photos (*A–C*). One-year postoperative photos (*D–F*).

taken 6 weeks after the procedures showing complete resolution of erythema by 6 weeks.

Case 5 (**Fig. 6**): Another case of concurrent treatment with full-face CO_2 laser resurfacing and facelift in a 59-year-old female. The Lumenis Ultrapulse CO_2 laser with the Deep FX handpiece attached was used to treat the perioral region with the following settings: 25 mJ, density 5%, 50% overlap. A single pass was made. The remainder of the face (except for that skin contained within the orbital rims) was treated at the following settings: 20 mJ, density 5%, 50% overlap. A single pass was made. Eschar was removed with saline-soaked gauze. The Active FX handpiece was then affixed to the laser and used to resurface the facial skin (except for the skin within the confines of the orbital rims) at the following settings: 100 mJ, 60W, pattern 1, size 9, density 6. Two passes were made in vertical

and horizontal painting patterns. Eschar was removed with saline-soaked gauze. For the skin within the confines of the orbital rims, a single pass was made at the following settings: 80 mJ, 40W, pattern 5, size 6, density 4. The postoperative photos were taken 1 year after the procedures.

Case 6 (**Fig. 7**): 70-year-old female status post concurrent full-face CO_2 laser resurfacing and facelift. Preop and postop photos were taken one year apart. At the completion of the facelift, the Lumenis Ultrapulse CO_2 laser was then brought into the field and the Active FX handpiece was attached. The first pass was performed on the lower eyelids (80 mJ, density 3, 45W). A second pass was made under the same settings. The central face including the forehead, nose, medial cheeks, and perioral region was then treated with three passes total (identical settings). The skin

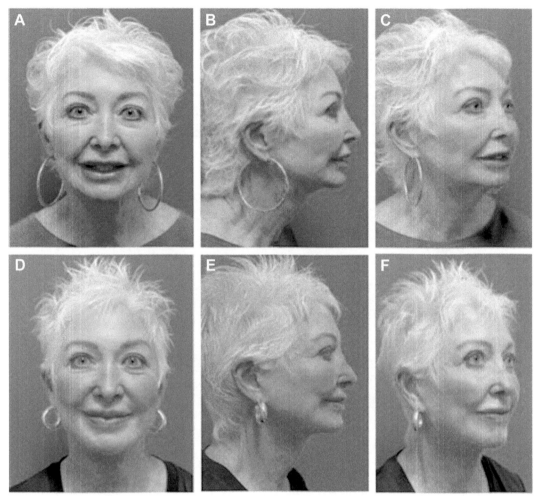

Fig. 7. Concurrent full-face CO$_2$ laser resurfacing and facelift in a 70-year-old female. Preoperative photos (A–C). One-year postoperative photos (D–F).

flaps were then treated with two passes in orthogonal painting patterns.

Case 7 (Fig. 8): In this case, a concurrent treatment of neck lift and full-face CO$_2$ laser resurfacing was performed in a 75-year-old female. Following the neck lift, the Lumenis Ultrapulse CO$_2$ laser was then brought into the field and the Active FX handpiece was attached. The first pass was performed on the lower eyelids (60 mJ, density 5, 45W). A second pass was made under the same settings. The central face including the forehead, nose, medial cheeks, and perioral region was then treated with three passes (identical settings). The skin flaps were then treated with two passes at 50 mJ, density 4, 45W. Postprocedure photos were taken at 1 year.

Case 8 (Fig. 9): This case shows impressive results (1-year postprocedure), in a 60-year-old female who underwent stand-alone full-face CO$_2$

skin resurfacing. The Lumenis Ultrapulse CO2 laser with the Deep FX handpiece attached was used to treat the perioral region with the following settings: 25 mJ, density 5%, 50% overlap. A single pass was made. The remainder of the face (except for that skin contained within the orbital rims) was treated at the following settings: 20 mJ, density 5%, 50% overlap. A single pass was made. Eschar was removed with saline-soaked gauze. The Active FX handpiece was then affixed to the laser and used to resurface the facial skin (except for the skin within the confines of the orbital rims) at the following settings: 100 mJ, 60W, pattern 1, size 9, density 6. Two nonoverlapping passes were made in vertical and horizontal painting patterns. Eschar was removed with saline-soaked gauze. For the skin within the confines of the orbital rims, a single pass was made at the following settings: 80 mJ, 40W, pattern 5, size 6, density 4.

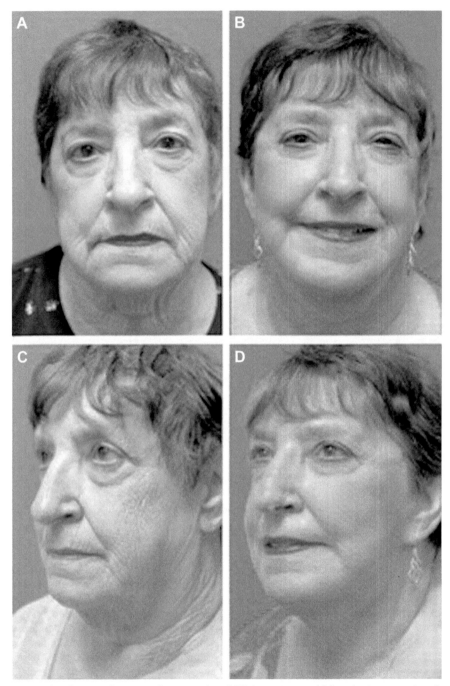

Fig. 8. Concurrent full-face CO_2 laser resurfacing and neck lift in a 75-year-old female. Preoperative photos (*A, C*). One-year postoperative photos (*B, D*).

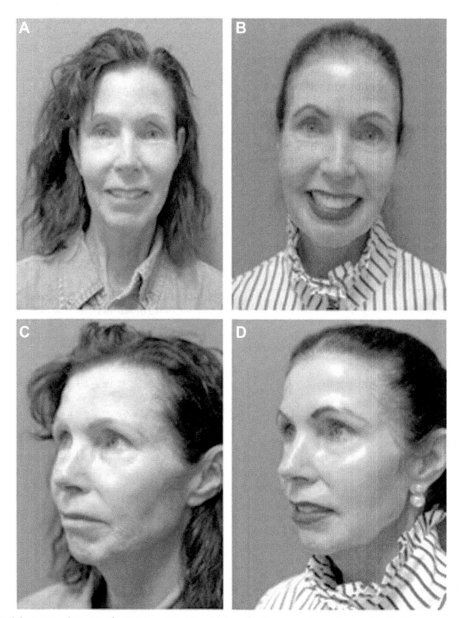

Fig. 9. Full-face CO_2 skin resurfacing in a 60-year-old female. Preprocedure photos (*A, C*). One-year postprocedure photos (*B, D*).

SUMMARY

Although many different technologies/techniques exist for facial and neck skin rejuvenation, fractionated CO_2 laser allows for significant skin tightening, reduction in rhytid burden, high patient satisfaction, and a manageable side effect/complication profile. This has been proven to be safe and effective in concurrent treatment with other aging face procedures such as rhytidectomy and endoscopic browlift. The optimal results are dependent on the operator's technique and experience and cannot be replaced by the use of laser technology.

CLINICS CARE POINTS

- The ideal candidates for laser skin resurfacing are patients with Fitzpatrick skin types I-II but

Fitzpatrick type III can also be considered for laser resurfacing (albeit less aggressively).

- In the senior author's practice, all patients are started on valacyclovir, fluconazole, and cephalexin one day prior to their treatment to decrease the potential risk of post-procedural herpetic, fungal, and bacterial infections but these treatments are controversial.

- Concurrent CO_2 laser resurfacing with other aging face procedures such as rhytidectomy should be considered as it has proven to be safe and can yield excellent results.

- The immediate endpoint in superficial CO_2 laser resurfacing is the removal of the epidermal layer of the skin and exposure of the papillary dermis that clinically is distinguishable with yellowing of the wound bed and pinpoint bleeding.

DISCLOSURE

The authors have no personal or financial conflicts of interest to disclose.

REFERENCES

1. Kitzmiller WJ, Visscher M, Page DA, et al. A controlled evaluation of dermabrasion versus CO2 laser resurfacing for the treatment of perioral wrinkles. Plast Reconstr Surg 2000;106(6):1366–72 [discussion: 1373-1364].
2. Reed JT, Joseph AK, Bridenstine JB. Treatment of periorbital wrinkles. A comparison of the SilkTouch carbon dioxide laser with a medium-depth chemical peel. Dermatol Surg 1997;23(8):643–8.
3. Altshuler GB, Anderson RR, Manstein D, et al. Extended theory of selective photothermolysis. Lasers Surg Med 2001;29(5):416–32.
4. Ross EV, Miller C, Meehan K, et al. One-pass CO2 versus multiple-pass Er:YAG laser resurfacing in the treatment of rhytides: a comparison side-by-side study of pulsed CO2 and Er:YAG lasers. Dermatol Surg 2001;27(8):709–15.
5. Hohenleutner S, Hohenleutner U, Landthaler M. Comparison of erbium: YAG and carbon dioxide laser for the treatment of facial rhytides. Arch Dermatol 1999;135(11):1416–7.
6. van Hillegersberg R. Fundamentals of laser surgery. Eur J Sur 1997;163(1):3–12.
7. Guttenberg SA, Emery RW 3rd. Laser physics and tissue interaction. Oral Maxill Surg Clin North Am 2004;16(2):143–7.
8. Gregory RO. Laser physics and physiology. Clin Plast Surg 1998;25(1):89–93.
9. Riggs K, Keller M, Humphreys TR. Ablative laser resurfacing: high-energy pulsed carbon dioxide and erbium:yttrium-aluminum-garnet. Clin Dermatol 2007;25(5):462–73.
10. Herd RM, Dover JS, Arndt KA. Basic laser principles. Dermatol Clin 1997;15(3):355–72.
11. Fisher JC. Basic biophysical principles of resurfacing of human skin by means of the carbon dioxide laser. J Clin Laser Med Surg 1996;14(4):193–210.
12. Polanyi TG. Physics of surgery with lasers. Clin Chest Med 1985;6(2):179–202.
13. Gillis TM, Strong MS. Surgical lasers and soft tissue interactions. Otolaryngol Clin North Am 1983;16(4):775–84.
14. Janda P, Sroka R, Mundweil B, et al. Comparison of thermal tissue effects induced by contact application of fiber guided laser systems. Lasers Surg Med 2003;33(2):93–101.
15. Absten GT. Physics of light and lasers. Obstet Gynecol Clin North Am 1991;18(3):407–27.
16. Reinisch L. Laser physics and tissue interactions. Otolaryngol Clin North Am 1996;29(6):893–914.
17. Ratz JL. Laser physics. Clin Dermatol 1995;13(1):11–20.
18. Moy RL, Bucalo B, Lee MH, et al. Skin resurfacing of facial rhytides and scars with the 90-microsecond short pulse CO2 laser. Comparison to the 900-microsecond dwell time CO2 lasers and clinical experience. Dermatol Surg 1998;24(12):1390–6.
19. Xu XG, Gao XH, Li YH, et al. Ultrapulse-mode versus superpulse-mode fractional carbon dioxide laser on normal back skin. Dermatol Surg 2013;39(7):1047–55.
20. Luo YJ, Xu XG, Wu Y, et al. Split-face comparison of ultrapulse-mode and superpulse-mode fractionated carbon dioxide lasers on photoaged skin. J Drugs Dermatol : JDD 2012;11(11):1310–4.
21. Trelles MA, Rigau J, Mellor TK, et al. A clinical and histological comparison of flashscanning versus pulsed technology in carbon dioxide laser facial skin resurfacing. Dermatol Surg 1998;24(1):43–9.
22. Orringer JS, Sachs DL, Shao Y, et al. Direct quantitative comparison of molecular responses in photodamaged human skin to fractionated and fully ablative carbon dioxide laser resurfacing. Dermatol Surg 2012;38(10):1668–77.
23. Sherry SD, Miles BA, Finn RA. Long-term efficacy of carbon dioxide laser resurfacing for facial actinic keratosis. J Oral Maxill Surg 2007;65(6):1135–9.
24. Borges J, Araújo L, Cuzzi T, et al. Fractional Laser Resurfacing Treats Photoaging by Promoting Neocollagenesis and Cutaneous Edema. J Clin Aesthet Dermatol 2020;13(1):22–7.
25. Baker DC. Lateral SMASectomy, plication and short scar facelifts: indications and techniques. Clin Plast Surg 2008;35(4):533–50, vi.

26. Glogau RG, Matarasso SL. Chemical face peeling: patient and peeling agent selection. Facial Plast Surg : FPS 1995;11(1):1–8.

27. Fitzpatrick TB. The validity and practicality of sun-reactive skin types I through VI. Arch Dermatol 1988;124(6):869–71.

28. Alexis AF. Lasers and light-based therapies in ethnic skin: treatment options and recommendations for Fitzpatrick skin types V and VI. Br J Dermatol 2013;169(Suppl 3):91–7.

29. Alster T, Hirsch R. Single-pass CO2 laser skin resurfacing of light and dark skin: extended experience with 52 patients. J Cosmet Laser Ther 2003;5(1):39–42.

30. Hamilton MM, Kao R. Recognizing and managing complications in laser resurfacing, chemical peels, and dermabrasion. Facial Plast Surg Clin North Am 2020;28(4):493–501.

31. Hunzeker CM, Weiss ET, Geronemus RG. Fractionated CO2 laser resurfacing: our experience with more than 2000 treatments. Aesthet Surg J 2009; 29(4):317–22.

32. Krupa Shankar D, Chakravarthi M, Shilpakar R. Carbon dioxide laser guidelines. J Cutan Aesthet Surg 2009;2(2):72–80.

33. Alexiades-Armenakas MR, Dover JS, Arndt KA. The spectrum of laser skin resurfacing: nonablative, fractional, and ablative laser resurfacing. J Am Acad Dermatol 2008;58(5):719–37 [quiz: 738-740].

34. Manuskiatti W, Fitzpatrick RE, Goldman MP. Long-term effectiveness and side effects of carbon dioxide laser resurfacing for photoaged facial skin. J Am Acad Dermatol 1999;40(3):401–11.

35. Campbell TM, Goldman MP. Adverse events of fractionated carbon dioxide laser: review of 373 treatments. Dermatol Surg 2010;36(11):1645–50.

36. Sriprachya-Anunt S, Fitzpatrick RE, Goldman MP, et al. Infections complicating pulsed carbon dioxide laser resurfacing for photoaged facial skin. Dermatol Surg 1997;23(7):527–35 [discussion: 535-526].

37. Manuskiatti W, Fitzpatrick RE, Goldman MP, et al. Prophylactic antibiotics in patients undergoing laser resurfacing of the skin. J Am Acad Dermatol 1999; 40(1):77–84.

38. Gaspar Z, Vinciullo C, Elliott T. Antibiotic prophylaxis for full-face laser resurfacing: is it necessary? Arch Dermatol 2001;137(3):313–5.

39. Alster TS, Lupton JR. Prevention and treatment of side effects and complications of cutaneous laser resurfacing. Plast Reconstr Surg 2002;109(1): 308–16 [discussion: 317-308].

40. Goldman MP. The use of hydroquinone with facial laser resurfacing. J Cutan Laser Ther 2000;2(2): 73–7.

41. Wong ITY, Richer V. Prophylaxis of post-inflammatory hyperpigmentation from energy-based device treatments: a review [Formula: see text]. J Cutan Med Surg 2021;25(1):77–86.

42. Kilmer SL, Chotzen V, Zelickson BD, et al. Full-face laser resurfacing using a supplemented topical anesthesia protocol. Arch Dermatol 2003;139(10): 1279–83.

43. Bjerring P, Andersen PH, Arendt-Nielsen L. Vascular response of human skin after analgesia with EMLA cream. Br J Anaesth 1989;63(6):655–60.

44. Naouri M, Atlan M, Perrodeau E, et al. High-resolution ultrasound imaging to demonstrate and predict efficacy of carbon dioxide fractional resurfacing laser treatment. Dermatol Surg 2011;37(5):596–603.

45. Altshuler GB, Zenzie HH, Erofeev AV, et al. Contact cooling of the skin. Phys Med Biol 1999;44(4): 1003–23.

46. Kelly KM, Nelson JS, Lask GP, et al. Cryogen spray cooling in combination with nonablative laser treatment of facial rhytides. Arch Dermatol 1999;135(6): 691–4.

47. Rohrich RJ, Gyimesi IM, Clark P, et al. CO2 laser safety considerations in facial skin resurfacing. Plast Reconstr Surg 1997;100(5):1285–90.

48. Wald D, Michelow BJ, Guyuron B, et al. Fire hazards and CO2 laser resurfacing. Plast Reconstr Surg 1998;101(1):185–8.

49. Hirshman CA, Smith J. Indirect ignitioin of the endotracheal tube during carbon dioxide laser surgery. Arch Otolaryngol 1980;106(10):639–41.

50. Fader DJ, Ratner D. Principles of CO2/erbium laser safety. Dermatol Surg 2000;26(3):235–9.

51. Kotlus BS. Dual-depth fractional carbon dioxide laser resurfacing for periocular rhytidosis. Dermatol Surg 2010;36(5):623–8.

52. Ramsdell WM. Fractional carbon dioxide laser resurfacing. Semin Plast Surg 2012;26(3):125–30.

53. Baker TJ. Chemical face peeling and rhytidectomy. A combined approach for facial rejuvenation. Plast Reconstr Surg Transplant Bull 1962;29:199–207.

54. Guyuron B, Michelow B, Schmelzer R, et al. Delayed healing of rhytidectomy flap resurfaced with CO2 laser. Plast Reconstr Surg 1998;101(3):816–9.

55. Park GC, Wiseman JB, Hayes DK. The evaluation of rhytidectomy flap healing after CO2 laser resurfacing in a pig model. Otolaryngol Head Neck Surg 2001;125(6):590–2.

56. Wright EJ, Struck SK. Facelift combined with simultaneous fractional laser resurfacing: Outcomes and complications. J Plast Reconstr Aesthet Surg 2015; 68(10):1332–7.

57. Truswell WHt. Combining fractional carbon-dioxide laser resurfacing with face-lift surgery. Facial Plast Surg Clin North Am 2012;20(2):201–13, vi.

58. Ramirez OM, Pozner JN. Laser resurfacing as an adjunct to endoforehead lift, endofacelift, and biplanar facelift. Ann Plast Surg 1997;38(4):315–21 [discussion: 321-312].

59. Koch BB, Perkins SW. Simultaneous rhytidectomy and full-face carbon dioxide laser resurfacing: a

case series and meta-analysis. Arch Facial Plast Surg 2002;4(4):227–33.

60. Li D, Lin SB, Cheng B. Complications and posttreatment care following invasive laser skin resurfacing: a review. J Cosmet Laser Ther 2018;20(3):168–78.

61. Fulton JE Jr. Complications of laser resurfacing. Methods of prevention and management. Dermatol Surg 1998;24(1):91–9.

62. Hirschmann JV. Antimicrobial prophylaxis in dermatology. Semin Cutan Med Surg 2000;19(1):2–9.

63. Nanni CA, Alster TS. Complications of cutaneous laser surgery. A Review Dermatol Surg 1998;24(2):209–19.

64. Franck P, Henderson PW, Rothaus KO. Basics of lasers: history, physics, and clinical Applications. Clin Plast Surg 2016;43(3):505–13.

Mastering Midface Injections

Hillary A. Newsome, MD, John J. Chi, MD, MPHS*

KEYWORDS

• Midface • Filler • Hyaluronic acid • Aging face • Nonsurgical facial rejuvenation

KEY POINTS

• The paradigm of the aging face has shifted from vertical descent of tissues to volume loss and pseudoptosis as the causes for the stigmata of aging
• Filler injection of the midface must respect certain anatomic considerations and focus on restoring lost volume
• Hyaluronic acid fillers are the most commonly used filler in the infraorbital hollow/tear trough and cheek regions

INTRODUCTION

According to the American Academy of Facial Plastic and Reconstructive Surgery filler injection was the second most common minimally invasive cosmetic procedure performed in 2020.[1] For the aging face, filler can be used as a stand-alone procedure or in conjunction with other treatment modalities. In the past several decades, improved knowledge of facial anatomy has changed the way we think about aging and has improved treatment strategies and aesthetic outcomes.[2,3] As technology has advanced, so, too, have the options for reversing aging. The midface serves as an ideal target for rejuvenation via injectables.

DEFINING THE MIDFACE

Successful management of the aging midface requires mastery of its anatomy. The midface refers to the area of the face from the lower eyelid to the oral commissure.[4] The superior border of the midface is the inferior periorbita and includes the lower lid–cheek junction, which has particular significance in midfacial rejuvenation. Medially, the boundary of the midface is the nose/pyriform aperture. It extends as far laterally as the helical root and tragus, as the zygomatic cheek.

Maintaining consistency with the neck and scalp, the midface is composed of 5 different layers: (1) skin (2) subcutaneous fat (3) superficial musculoaponeurotic system (SMAS) (4) deep fat tissue (5) periosteum.[5,6] It is worth noting the thickness of these layers varies, with there being little to no subcutaneous tissue in the lower lid region compared with the abundance of fat in the malar cheek. The bony structure is formed by the maxilla and zygoma/zygomatic arch.

Anatomy of the Facial Fat Compartments

There are 2 layers of fat compartments in the midface that are separated by the SMAS: the superficial and deep compartments. Each of these compartments is further subdivided. The superficial fat compartments are separated by fibrous septa.[7,8] The superficial fat compartments of the midface include (from medial to lateral): nasolabial fat, medial fat, middle fat, lateral temporal cheek fat.[8] (Fig. 1).[9] The terms "malar fat pad" and "cheek fat" most commonly refer to the superficial medial fat pad with the possible inclusion of the nasolabial and middle pads.[5,10] The medial and middle cheek compartments are separated by the middle cheek septum which is a dense fibrous barrier with a dermal insertion.[7] The inferior orbital fat pad lies superior to the cheek fat and has a

Division of Facial Plastic & Reconstructive Surgery, Washington University Facial Plastic Surgery Center, Washington University in St. Louis-School of Medicine, 660 S Euclid AveCampus Box 8115St. Louis, MO 63110, USA
* Corresponding author.
E-mail address: Johnchi@wustl.edu

Facial Plast Surg Clin N Am 30 (2022) 347–356
https://doi.org/10.1016/j.fsc.2022.03.008
1064-7406/22/Published by Elsevier Inc.

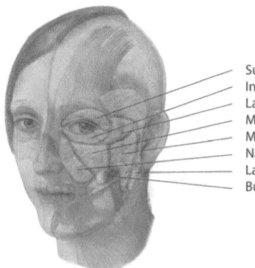

Superior orbital fat
Inferior orbital fat
Lateral orbital fat
Medial cheek fat
Middle cheek fat
Nasolabial fat
Lateral temporal-cheek fat
Buccal extension of the buccal fat

Fig. 1. The superficial fat pads of the midface. (*From* Gierloff M, Stohring C, Buder T, Gassling V, Acil Y, Wiltfang J. Aging changes of the midfacial fat compartments: a computed tomographic study. Plast Reconstr Surg. 2012;129(1):263-273.[9])

corresponding superior orbital fat pad. The fat of the deep compartment acts as the scaffold of the midface and many of the stigmata of an aging face are related to changes in this layer.[2,11] The deep layer includes the deep medial cheek fat, buccal fat, and lateral deep suborbicularis oculi fat (SOOF; **Fig. 2**).[9] The most relevant fat pads for the youthful midface are the deep medial cheek fat and SOOF, the latter of which is often broken up into medial and lateral SOOF.[2,12]

The deep medial cheek fat is a triangular compartment of fat that sits atop the maxilla. The compartment is bound medially by the ligaments

of the pyriform aperture, laterally by the zygomaticus major muscle, superiorly by the orbicularis retaining ligament, and the suborbicularis oris fat inferiorly.[2] The deep medial cheek fat receives it blood supply predominantly from the infraorbital artery and minor contributions from branches of the angular artery.

The medial portion of the SOOF begins at the medial limbus and extends to the lateral canthus. The deep medial cheek fat binds it medially. The lateral portion starts at the lateral canthus and extends to the temporal fat pad. Its superior border is the lateral orbital thickening/orbitomalar ligament

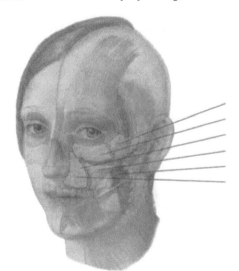

Sub–orbicularis oculi fat (lateral part)
Sub–orbicularis oculi fat (medial part)
Deep medial cheek fat (medial part)
Deep medial cheek fat (lateral part)
Buccal extension of the buccal fat
Ristow´s space

Fig. 2. The deep fat pads of the midface. (*From* Gierloff M, Stohring C, Buder T, Gassling V, Acil Y, Wiltfang J. Aging changes of the midfacial fat compartments: a computed tomographic study. Plast Reconstr Surg. 2012;129(1):263-273.[9])

and the inferior border is the zygomaticocutaneous ligament.[13] The buccal fat pad extends from the buccinator to the temporal space, and its depth varies. It is typically noted to have multiple components including buccal, pterygoid, superficial, and temporal limbs.[14,15]

THE AGING MIDFACE

- Characteristics of midfacial aging include: loss of a smooth transition between the lower lid and cheek, appearance of a double convexity of the cheek, and prominent melolabial folds
- All layers of the face experience changes with aging

The hallmark of midfacial aging includes several notable characteristics that should be identified on patient examination. There is disruption of a smooth lower lid–cheek junction. The Ogee curve can be lost and a double convexity (from lateral view) may appear. This results from a greater weakening of the orbitomalar ligament compared with the zygomaticocutaneous ligament, creating a tear trough and malar mound.[16,17] The loss of anterior projection and fullness of the malar region that can be seen is a result of both bony and soft tissue changes causing a deepening of the melolabial fold.

The structure of the midface is largely reliant on the volume and position of the deep fat and the bony structure, on which it sits atop. Nearly all layers of the face experience changes with aging. The bony structure of the face is well known to be affected by resorption.[18] In particular, the orbital aperture undergoes enlargement and contributes to the hollowed appearance of the periorbita. Additionally, the overall height and projection of the maxilla have been found to decrease.[19,20]

The soft tissue experiences aging as well. Initially, changes were thought to be secondary to gravity and descent of tissue, but more recently, volume loss in critical areas has been identified as the predominant contributor to the appearance of an aged midface.[3] The prominence of soft tissue grooves like the "tear trough" and heavy melolabial folds that are seen with aging may be explained by the "pseudoptosis" theory. "Pseudoptosis" refers to the volumetric depletion of the midfacial fat compartments and a resulting loss of anterior projection of the cheek. Excess facial skin (due to the volume decrease), in turn, creates a prominent melolabial fold.[2] The fat pads of the midface have been shown in several imaging and even histologic studies to have changing morphology with age.[9,21] **Fig. 3** shows an aged and deflated midface with prominent melolabial fold that improves with the injection of saline into the deep medial cheek compartment.[2]

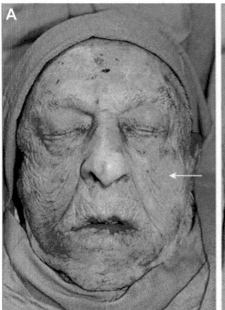 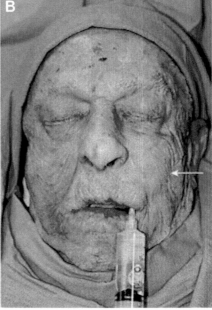

Fig. 3. (A) An aged and deflated midface with prominent melolabial fold that improves with (B) injection of saline into the deep medial cheek compartment (cadaveric specimen). (From Rohrich RJ, Pessa JE, Ristow B. The youthful cheek and the deep medial fat compartment. Plast Reconstr Surg. 2008;121(6):2107-2112.[2])

Importantly, the skin also displays changes. The epidermis and dermis experience thinning, and the ratio of collagen type III to type I increases.[22,23] These changes result in increased skin laxity and decreased resiliency.[24] Dyschromias become more prevalent and the skin tone becomes uneven. Photoaging can also cause significant differences in skin appearance.[25]

REJUVENATION OF THE MIDFACE WITH INJECTABLE FILLER

Increasing in popularity, rejuvenation of the midface with injectable filler has been shown to be an effective means of restoring lost midfacial volume. The nuances of this technique include knowing which type of filler to use for a given site and where/how to deposit it.

The scientific properties of fillers have been heavily investigated, resulting in the creation of fillers with unique characteristics. While an in-depth discussion of the mechanical properties of injectables is beyond the scope of this review, some basic information is necessary to choose the best-suited injection material for a desirable outcome. The modulus of elasticity (G′) represents a substances' ability to withstand deformation. Materials with a higher G′ are stiffer and less malleable compared with products with a lower G′. Changes in G′ are determined by the type of material, as well as specific properties such as cross-linking and particle size.[26] Lower G′ fillers are indicated for superficial rhytids such as the under-eye area, whereas firmer materials can be used in the lower midface. Materials that are more hydrophilic will absorb water and potentially cause swelling and spread of the injected material.

The most commonly used filler used for minimally invasive cosmetic procedures in 2020 was hyaluronic acid and its derivatives.[27] This includes the Juvéderm (Allergan Inc.; Irvine, CA) family of injectable gel fillers, of which there are currently 5 different preparations; Belotero (Merz Pharma GmbH; Frankfurt, Germany); and the Restylane line of gel fillers with 7 different formulations (Galderma Laboratories; Fort Worth, Texas). Nonhyaluronic acid fillers are less common, but still frequently used, and include calcium hydroxylapatite like Radiesse (Merz North America; Franksville, Wisconsin) and poly-L-lactic acid like Sculptra Aesthetic (Galderma Laboratories; Fort Worth, Texas). The injection technique and layer of deposition may change depending on which filler is used. Once the filler type has been selected, the method of injection is largely up to the provider. Depending on the material, depth, and location of placement, fillers can last from 6 to 24 months.[28]

Before injection, many providers choose to anesthetize the skin with topical anesthetic lidocaine/benzocaine preparations or pretreat the area with ice packs. Another option for pain control is to perform local blocks of the infraorbital and zygomaticofacial nerves. Care must be taken though, to use a sufficiently small local anesthetic bolus so as to not disturb the overlying tissue contour.[5] Additionally, many newer generation fillers contain lidocaine and anesthetize as the filler injection is carried out. To lessen the discomfort during injection, vibrating devices have also been used to minimize the effects of noxious stimuli.[29] Immediately before injection, the skin should be cleansed. Options for prepping include isopropyl alcohol, chlorhexidine, and providone-iodine.

The two methods of delivery include the use of a needle, versus the use of a blunt-tipped cannula, to deposit the filler. Fillers typically come prepackaged with needles only, so blunt-tipped cannulas need to be purchased separately. For introduction into the skin, a scalpel or a needle 1 to 2 sizes larger than the cannula can be used to create the skin opening before inserting the cannula. This step is mitigated with the technique of needle injection.

The use of a cannula has become preferred by many, as it is thought to be less traumatic maneuvering through tissue, theoretically creating less tissue injury and perhaps less bruising.[5,30] Proponents of this technique often report less chance of intravascular injection. Overall, there are extremely low rates of intravascular injection for both needle and cannula delivery.[31] Before injection with either method, it is recommended to retract the plunger to create and aspirating force.[5] If blood is aspirated at that time, intravascular injection may occur and injection in that location is not recommended. It is important to note, however, that this does not ensure the injection will not be intravascular, as the needle tip/cannula tip may change position during the aspiration and ensuing injection. A false negative aspiration can happen as well, for example, if vessel wall is being contacted.[31] Anterograde or retrograde deposition can be utilized.[32] Retrograde deposition is preferred, however, because it allows the injector to have improved tactile feedback regarding the injection force. If significant resistance is encountered, the needle/cannula tip may be in a tight tissue compartment or intravascular placement has occurred, and injection should not proceed.

Injection Technique for Infraorbital Hollows/ Tear Trough

- The tear trough region has little subcutaneous fat and very thin overlying tissue

- The Tyndall effect (bluish hue seen through the skin) can occur in this area
- Injectors must recognize the location of the infraorbital foramen and angular artery
- Injection end point is the restoration of smoother lower lid–cheek junction
- Providers should correctly identify patients suffering from fat herniation/lower lid bags that will not improve with filler injection

This area can be treated with either needle or cannula with acceptable results. Entry point for blunt-tipped cannula injection can be in the midline cheek tissue below the inferior orbital rim. In one published clinical approach summary, selecting an entry point in the thicker tissue of the cheek was thought to minimize the bruising that can occur when injecting directly into the thinner tissue of the lower eyelid. This location still allows access to both the lower lid and cheek.[5]

Filler in this region is most commonly deposited just above the periosteum for higher G′ materials, and subcutaneously for lower G′ products. Deeper injections, also termed vertical supra/preperiosteal technique, can be delivered just beneath the orbital rim, several millimeters apart.[32] Filler placed here helps restore the youthful contour of the lower lid–cheek junction.[33] It is worthwhile to note that the SOOF has been shown to experience the greatest correlation between tissue response and volume of filler injected.[12] Injectors should be aware of the infraorbital neurovascular bundle in the midpupillary line and the angular artery located more medially.

More superficial injections in this region can also be used. For these, many injectors use a linear threading or fanning motion to deposit the filler in the subcutaneous or submuscular plane. The thin skin of this region can cause a bluish discoloration (Tyndall effect) and can create visible contour irregularities.[5,33] (Fig. 4C).[34] Should visible or palpable irregularities arise, these can be smoothed out with gentle palpation.[32] Because of the hydrophilic nature of hyaluronic fillers, some advocate for the dilution of filler in this area with either lidocaine or saline to minimize postprocedural edema.[34] It is important to note, however, postproduction manipulation of hyaluronic acid fillers may yield a heterogeneous injectable.[35] Fig. 4B depicts the endpoint of injection.[34]

Injection Technique for Cheek

- Three to 5 injection locations along the zygoma are preferred over a single injection site
- Injection endpoint is improved anterior projection of the cheek and softening of the melolabial folds
- Providers should check the smile frequently to prevent overfilling of the cheek
- Injectors must note the location of the angular artery when addressing the melolabial fold

The medial and lateral cheek and lower midface can all undergo volume restoration with filler. Again, both cannula techniques and needles can

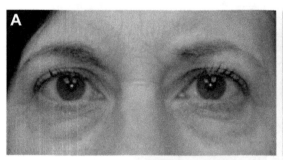
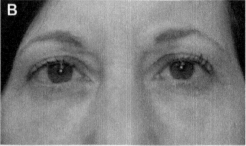
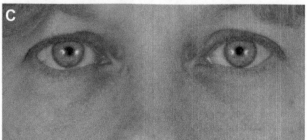

Fig. 4. (A,B) Before and after hyaluronic acid filler injection of the tear trough (superficial) and orbital rim (deep). (C) Blue discoloration of the infraorbital region due to the Tyndall effect. (From Tan M, Kontis TC. Midface volumization with injectable fillers. Facial Plast Surg Clin North Am. 2015;23(2):233-242.[34])

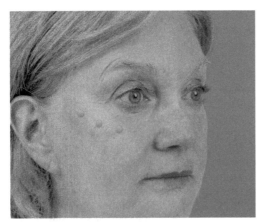

Fig. 5. Potential injection sites for the cheek are shown. Typically, 3 to 5 locations are used and filler is deposited preperiosteally. Here, 3 injection points along the cheek are depicted: (1) in-line with the lateral canthus, (2) malar eminence, (3) midpoint of the zygomatic arch.

be successful in this area. Most injectors recommend a high G′ filler.[32–34,36–38] The stiffer nature of these materials allows for the support necessary to lift the overlying tissue with a durable response. Autologous fat injection is also an option in this area.

Preperiosteal depot techniques typically use 3 to 5 depot locations spanning anteromedially

from the malar eminence and moving laterally along the zygoma and zygomatic arch.[36] Using multiple injection locations that respect the cheek subunits results in a more natural restoration than a single injection point would yield.[5] **Fig. 5** depicts potential injection locations. It is helpful to recognize the superolateral quadrant of the cheek should have the most volume.[39]

During injection, it is important to assess the patient at rest and with smiling because overfilling can occur and result in an unnatural appearance of the cheek during animation.[5,40] Injectors should avoid the tendency to want to continue to add filler to the deep medial cheek compartment given its low surface-volume coefficient and must assess the smile before adding additional filler.[12] Stopping point is determined when the folds and shadows have softened and the midface has been lifted.[5,41] (**Fig. 6**).[41] Some injectors are proponents of injecting the medial and lateral cheek before the injection of the tear trough; because as the volume is restored and folds are effaced, sometimes a smaller amount of filler is required to address the tear trough.[5,33]

For the treatment of the melolabial fold, filler may be deposited into a subdermal plane using linear threading cross-hatching, fanning, or tower technique to slowly efface the fold. Entry point for cannula can be just lateral to the oral

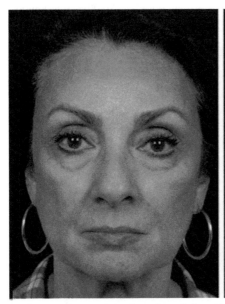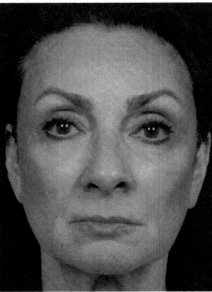

Fig. 6. This patient underwent injection of medial and lateral SOOF with hyaluronic acid filler and 25g cannula, as well as the deep medial and lateral cheek compartments with calcium hydroxlyapatite and 25g cannula. Notice the improvement of her tear trough and the melolabial folds. (*Reprinted from* Fitzgerald R. Addressing Facial Shape and Proportions with Injectable Agents in Youth and Age. In: Azizzadeh BM, MR; Johnson, CM; Massry, GG; Fitzgerald, R, ed. Master Techniques in Facial Rejuvenation. 2nd ed: Elsevier; 2018:15-54. © 2018 with permission from Elsevier.[41])

commissure. Entry here also allows access to the marionette lines (**Fig. 7**).[42] Injectors should be aware of the location of the angular artery.

Complications and Pitfalls

The spectrum of complications from filler injection ranges from minor and temporary, to permanent and organ threatening. The most common complications of filler injection include pain at the injection site, which can be mediated with local blocks, mixture of lidocaine, topical anesthetics, and vibratory devices as previously discussed.[5,29,33] Pain is usually short lived during the injection process, while ongoing discomfort may be a more ominous sign. Knowledge of the underlying vascular network and use of a blunt-tipped cannula and posttreatment ice can lessen the chance of bruising. It is important to note and counsel patients that some areas, such as the infraorbital hollow, are more prone to bruising (**Fig. 8A**).[42] Additionally, it is not uncommon for patients to experience edema, the severity of which can be affected by the filler's properties.

One complication, known as the Tyndall effect—a notable bluish discoloration of areas whereby hyaluronic acid filler has been placed—is widely described.[26,33,43] This is a result of the filler particles changing light refraction in areas of thin skin. Careful preoperative assessment should also evaluate for the Tyndall effect in a patient who may have been treated previously. Hyaluronidase (a natural occurring enzyme that breaks down hyaluronic acid) can be injected into the area, followed by massage to dissolve the particles with improvement in the color change over the next several days.[43]

The reversible nature of hyaluronic acid fillers with hyaluronidase has likely contributed to its popularity. For example, should a patient return with palpable nodules from poor distribution of product or simply have a change in heart, hyaluronic acid fillers can be dissolved. Other filler materials such as calcium hydroxylapatite do not carry this same benefit.

The most dreaded complication of filler injection is intravascular injection leading to skin necrosis or blindness. It is important to note, however, that extravascular compression, in addition to emboli, can similarly result compromised blood supply.[44] The vascular network can be identified by imaging devices to help minimize the risk.[44,45] The signs of skin necrosis begin to declare themselves immediately with blanching and pain in the area fed by the affected vessel. Should these signs be noted, immediate cessation of injection is warranted

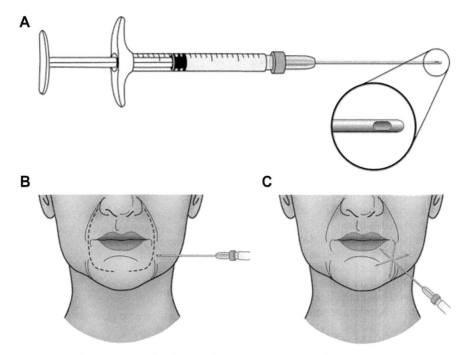

Fig. 7. (*A*) Blunt-tipped cannula. (*B, C*)Technique for injection subdermally with a fanning motion via blunt-tipped cannula is depicted for the marionette lines. Melolabial folds can be accessed through this site if cannula is long enough, or entry point lateral to the oral commissure can be used. (*From* Alam M, Tung R. Injection technique in neurotoxins and fillers: Indications, products, and outcomes. J Am Acad Dermatol. 2018;79(3):423-435.[42])

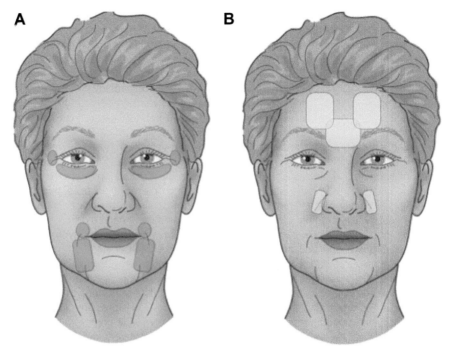

Fig. 8. (A) Regions of the face commonly affected by bruising after filler insertion. (B) High-risk regions for intravascular injection due to the supratrochlear and angular arteries. (*From* Alam M, Tung R. Injection technique in neurotoxins and fillers: Indications, products, and outcomes. J Am Acad Dermatol. 2018;79(3):423-435.[42])

followed by massage, warm compresses, injection of hyaluronidase, and application of topical nitroglycerin paste (for vasodilation).[5,43] Immediate debridement is not indicated, as the extent of skin necrosis is not always apparent initially. Necrosis can also result from extravascular compression.[44] Blindness is thought to occur from retrograde flow of emboli to the vascular supply of the eye. Injection into the nose, glabella, and forehead are the most common injection locations associated with vision loss.[46] Fig. 8B depicts high-risk regions for intravascular injection.[42]

DISCUSSION

Injectable fillers offer a minimally invasive technique for midfacial rejuvenation. Deflation of the deep fat compartments of the midface creates the characteristic hollows and deepening folds of an aging face. Filler injection can help recontour the lower lid–cheek junction and return the lost bulk of the midface. Hyaluronic acid fillers are a popular choice among injectors because of the variety of preparations available, and their reversibility. Each patient requires careful assessment to identify target areas for an optimal aesthetic outcome. Knowledge of the underlying anatomy and careful injection technique is critical to preventing serious complications and poor outcomes.

CLINICS CARE POINTS

- The paradigm of the aging face has shifted from vertical descent of tissues to volume loss and pseudoptosis as the causes for the stigmata of aging
- Knowledge of the anatomy of the fat compartments of the midface is critical to providing and an acceptable outcome
- The most common targets for filler injection of the midface are the infraorbital hollow/tear trough, the anterior cheek, and the melolabial fold
- Filler complications can range from minor to organ threatening and are avoided by proper technique

DISCLOSURE

The authors have no conflicts of interest or disclosures to report.

REFERENCES

1. AAFPRS Announce Annual Survey Results. A Look at How COVID-19 Disrupted Facial Plastic Surgery

and Aesthetics. 2021. Available at: https://www.
aafprs.org/Media/Press_Releases/PageTemplates/
NewSurveyResultsAnnouncedFeb.1,2021.aspx. Accessed November 1, 2021.

2. Rohrich RJ, Pessa JE, Ristow B. The youthful cheek
and the deep medial fat compartment. Plast Reconstr Surg 2008;121(6):2107–12.

3. Lambros V. Models of facial aging and implications
for treatment. Clin Plast Surg 2008;35(3):319–27.

4. Chi JJ. Periorbital Surgery: Forehead, Brow, and
Midface. Facial Plast Surg Clin North Am 2016;
24(2):107–17.

5. Cotofana S, Schenck TL, Trevidic P, et al. Midface:
Clinical Anatomy and Regional Approaches with
Injectable Fillers. Plast Reconstr Surg 2015;136(5
Suppl):219S–34S.

6. Kruglikov I, Trujillo O, Kristen Q, et al. The Facial Adipose Tissue: A Revision. Facial Plast Surg 2016;
32(6):671–82.

7. Rohrich RJ, Pessa JE. The retaining system of the
face: histologic evaluation of the septal boundaries
of the subcutaneous fat compartments. Plast Reconstr Surg 2008;121(5):1804–9.

8. Rohrich RJ, Pessa JE. The fat compartments of the
face: anatomy and clinical implications for cosmetic
surgery. Plast Reconstr Surg 2007;119(7):2219–27.

9. Gierloff M, Stohring C, Buder T, et al. Aging changes
of the midfacial fat compartments: a computed
tomographic study. Plast Reconstr Surg 2012;
129(1):263–73.

10. Wan D, Amirlak B, Rohrich R, et al. The clinical
importance of the fat compartments in midfacial aging. Plast Reconstr Surg Glob Open 2013;1(9):e92.

11. Rohrich RJ, Avashia YJ, Savetsky IL. Prediction of
Facial Aging Using the Facial Fat Compartments.
Plast Reconstr Surg 2021;147(1S-2):38S–42S.

12. Cotofana S, Koban KC, Konstantin F, et al. The
Surface-Volume Coefficient of the Superficial and
Deep Facial Fat Compartments: A Cadaveric
Three-Dimensional Volumetric Analysis. Plast Re-
constr Surg 2019;143(6):1605–13.

13. Rohrich RJ, Arbique GM, Wong C, et al. The anatomy of suborbicularis fat: implications for periorbital
rejuvenation. Plast Reconstr Surg 2000;124(3).
946–51.

14. Stuzin JM, Wagstrom L, Kawamoto HK, et al. The
anatomy and clinical applications of the buccal fat
pad. Plast Reconstr Surg 1990;85(1):29–37.

15. Rohrich RJ, Stuzin JM, Savetsky IL, et al. The Role of
the Buccal Fat Pad in Facial Aesthetic Surgery. Plast
Reconstr Surg 2021;148(2):334–8.

16. Espinoza GM, Holds JB. Evaluation and treatment of
the tear trough deformity in lower blepharoplasty.
Semin Plast Surg 2007;21(1):57–64.

17. Mendelson BC, Muzaffar AR, Adams WP Jr. Surgical
anatomy of the midcheek and malar mounds. Plast
Reconstr Surg 2002;110(3):885–96.

18. Kahn DM, Shaw RB Jr. Aging of the bony orbit: a
three-dimensional computed tomographic study.
Aesthet Surg J 2008;28(3):258–64.

19. Cotofana S, Gotkin RH, Frank K, et al. The Functional
Anatomy of the Deep Facial Fat Compartments: A
Detailed Imaging-Based Investigation. Plast Re-
constr Surg 2019;143(1):53–63.

20. Pessa JE. An algorithm of facial aging: verification of
Lambros's theory by three-dimensional stereolithog-
raphy, with reference to the pathogenesis of midfacial aging, scleral show, and the lateral suborbital
trough deformity. Plast Reconstr Surg 2000;106(2):
479–88.

21. Wan D, Amirlak B, Giessler P, et al. The differing
adipocyte morphologies of deep versus superficial
midfacial fat compartments: a cadaveric study. Plast
Reconstr Surg 2014;133(5):615e–22e.

22. Montagna W, Carlisle K. Structural changes in aging
human skin. J Invest Dermatol 1979;73(1):47–53.

23. Lovell CR, Smolenski KA, Duance VC, et al. Type I
and III collagen content and fibre distribution in
normal human skin during ageing. Br J Dermatol
1987;117(4):419–28.

24. Langton AK, Graham HK, Griffiths CEM, et al.
Ageing significantly impacts the biomechanical
function and structural composition of skin. Exp Dermatol 2019;28(8):981–4.

25. Zouboulis CC, Ganceviciene R, Liakou AI, et al.
Aesthetic aspects of skin aging, prevention, and
local treatment. Clin Dermatol 2019;37(4):365–72.

26. Attenello NH, Maas CS. Injectable fillers: review of
material and properties. Facial Plast Surg 2015;
31(1):29–34.

27. American Society of Plastic Surgeons. Plastic Surgery Statistics. 2020. Available at: https://www.
plasticsurgery.org/documents/News/Statistics/2020/
plastic-surgery-statistics-full-report-2020.pdf. Accessed Steptember 28, 2021.

28. Few J, Cox SE, Paradkar-Mitragotri D, et al.
A Multicenter, Single-Blind Randomized, Controlled
Study of a Volumizing Hyaluronic Acid Filler for Midface Volume Deficit: Patient-Reported Outcomes at
2 Years. Aesthet Surg J 2015;35(5):580 00.

29. Kuwahara H, Ogawa R. Using a Vibration Device to
Ease Pain During Facial Needling and Injection.
Eplasty 2016;16:e9.

30. Niamtu J 3rd. Accurate and anatomic midface filler
injection by using cheek implants as an injection
template. Dermatol Surg 2008;34(1):93–5.

31. Alam M, Kakar R, Dover JS, et al. Rates of Vascular
Occlusion Associated With Using Needles vs Cannulas for Filler Injection. JAMA Dermatol 2021;
157(2):174–80.

32. Carruthers J, Rzany B, Sattler G, et al. Anatomic
guidelines for augmentation of the cheek and infraorbital hollow. Dermatol Surg 2012;38(7 Pt 2):
1223–33.

33. Kontis TC, Bunin L, Fitzgerald R. Injectable Fillers: Panel Discussion, Controversies, and Techniques. Facial Plast Surg Clin North Am 2018;26(2):225–36.

34. Tan M, Kontis TC. Midface volumization with injectable fillers. Facial Plast Surg Clin North Am 2015; 23(2):233–42.

35. Goldman MP, Few J, Binauld S, et al. Evaluation of Physicochemical Properties Following Syringe-to-Syringe Mixing of Hyaluronic Acid Dermal Fillers. Dermatol Surg 2020;46(12):1606–12.

36. de Maio M, DeBoulle K, Braz A, et al. Alliance for the Future of Aesthetics Consensus C. Facial Assessment and Injection Guide for Botulinum Toxin and Injectable Hyaluronic Acid Fillers: Focus on the Midface. Plast Reconstr Surg 2017;140(4):540e–50e.

37. Graivier MH, Bass LS, Busso M, et al. Calcium hydroxylapatite (Radiesse) for correction of the mid- and lower face: consensus recommendations. Plast Reconstr Surg 2007;120(6 Suppl):55S–66S.

38. Ramanadham SR, Rohrich RJ. Newer Understanding of Specific Anatomic Targets in the Aging Face as Applied to Injectables: Superficial and Deep Facial Fat Compartments–An Evolving Target for Site-Specific Facial Augmentation. Plast Reconstr Surg 2015;136(5 Suppl):49S–55S.

39. Hinderer UT. Malar implants for improvement of the facial appearance. Plast Reconstr Surg 1975;56(2): 157–65.

40. Cotofana S, Gotkin RH, Frank K, et al. Anatomy Behind the Facial Overfilled Syndrome: The Transverse Facial Septum. Dermatol Surg 2020;46(8): e16–22.

41. Fitzgerald R. Addressing Facial Shape and Proportions with Injectable Agents in Youth and Age. In: Azizzadeh BM MR, Johnson CM, Massry GG, et al, editors. Master techniques in facial rejuvenation. 2nd edition. Elsevier; 2018. p. 15–54.

42. Alam M, Tung R. Injection technique in neurotoxins and fillers: Indications, products, and outcomes. J Am Acad Dermatol 2018;79(3):423–35.

43. Nettar K, Maas C. Facial filler and neurotoxin complications. Facial Plast Surg 2012;28(3):288–93.

44. Lima VGF, Regattieri NAT, Pompeu MF, et al. External vascular compression by hyaluronic acid filler documented with high-frequency ultrasound. J Cosmet Dermatol 2019;18(6):1629–31.

45. Lee W, Oh W, Hong GW, et al. Novel technique of filler injection in the temple area using the vein detection device. J Plast Reconstr Aesthet Surg 2019;72(2):335–54.

46. Sorensen EP, Council ML. Update in Soft-Tissue Filler-Associated Blindness. Dermatol Surg 2020; 46(5):671–7.

Liquid Rhinoplasty

Noah Saad, MD[c], Christian L. Stallworth, MD[a,b],*

KEYWORDS

• Rhinoplasty • Nose • Injection • Filler • Hyaluronic acid • Noninvasive

KEY POINTS

• Liquid rhinoplasty has seen an increase in popularity over the last decade.
• Liquid rhinoplasty has diverse applications ranging from the primary treatment of nasal contours for improved aesthetic lines to the treatment of postsurgical contour irregularities, treatment of the poor surgical candidate, and even correction of acquired nasal deformities resulting from trauma or medical illness.
• Though less invasive than surgery, liquid rhinoplasty is not without substantial potential risk. Knowledge of complex soft tissue and vascular anatomy of the nasal envelope is paramount.

LIQUID RHINOPLASTY

The popularity of "liquid", or nonsurgical, rhinoplasty has grown considerably among both patients and surgeons over the last decade. Circa 2010, it was not uncommon at international rhinoplasty meetings to hear renowned rhinoplasty experts pan the idea of nasal injections. Furthermore, many staunchly argued that such a procedure being "non-surgical" eliminated its classification as rhinoplasty altogether. Nonetheless, counterarguments were equally strong in their support of any procedure altering the shape of the nose being deemed "rhino-" and "-plasty." Our goal here is not to argue the semantics of this debate, but rather to illustrate the technical highlights, indications, and limitations of this procedure.

Since 2019, rhinoplasty has been the most common cosmetic procedure performed in the United States, accounting for just more than 15% of all invasive cosmetic procedures.[1,2] Additionally, soft tissue filler injections were the second most common noninvasive cosmetic procedure performed in 2020, representing roughly 26% of all noninvasive procedures. Further, fillers using hyaluronic acid (HA) accounted for almost 77% of all soft tissue filler injections.[1] As techniques and technologies have evolved, so too have the popularity of minimally invasive cosmetic procedures, increasing from 11 million cases in 2010 to more than 15 million cases in 2020.[1,3] As we have gained knowledge, control, and experience with different fillers, we similarly have been able to diversify the applications and facial subsites injected with greater success and outcomes.

The earliest documentation of nonsurgical rhinoplasty came in 2006 when Beer described the use of filler augmentation in cases of nasal reconstruction after trauma or in cases of prior rhinoplasty.[4] Since that time, numerous descriptions of technique and application have grown in tandem along with the increasing popularity of nonsurgical rhinoplasty procedures.[5–11] Although nasal injections remain an "off-label" use in the United States, HA fillers have gained multiple applications for the nose. These include, but are not limited to, leveling a dorsal hump through the addition of volume above and below the dorsal convexity, filling of visible nasal concavities,

a Division of Facial Plastic and Reconstructive Surgery, Department of Otolaryngology – Head & Neck Surgery, Joe R. and Teresa Lozano Long School of Medicine UT Health San Antonio, 7703 Floyd Curl Dr. Mail Code 7777, San Antonio, TX 78229, USA; b Texas Plastic Surgery, 21 Spurs Lane, Suite 120, San Antonio, TX 78240, USA; c Division of Plastic and Reconstructive Surgery, Department of Surgery, Joe R. and Teresa Lozano Long School of Medicine UT Health San Antonio, 7703 Floyd Curl Drive, San Antonio, TX 78229, USA
* Corresponding author. Division of Facial Plastic and Reconstructive Surgery, Department of Otolaryngology – Head & Neck Surgery, Joe R. and Teresa Lozano Long School of Medicine UT Health San Antonio, 7703 Floyd Curl Dr. Mail Code 7777, San Antonio, TX 78229.
E-mail address: stallworth@uthscsa.edu

Facial Plast Surg Clin N Am 30 (2022) 357–364
https://doi.org/10.1016/j.fsc.2022.03.009
1064-7406/22/© 2022 Elsevier Inc. All rights reserved.

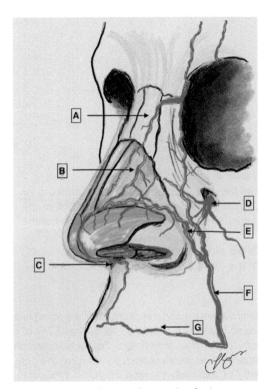

Fig. 1. Nasal vasculature. The nasal soft tissue enve-lope is supplied by both the internal and external ca-rotid arterial systems. Arteries are typically paired through anatomic variations with a single dominant dorsal nasal and/or columellar artery have been described. (A)- Dorsal nasal artery; (B) – external branch of the anterior ethmoid artery; (C)- columellar artery; (D)- infraorbital artery; (E)- lateral nasal artery; (F)- angular artery; (G)- superior labial artery.

correcting upper and middle third asymmetries, as well as improving the under-rotated or under pro-jected tip.[7,8] The entire dorsum can also be augmented to build up a profile in patients who have an underdeveloped bony and cartilaginous nasal skeleton.

NASAL ANATOMY

Before performing nonsurgical rhinoplasty, the surgeon must have a sound knowledge of the anatomy of the nose.[12–14] The layers of the nose include the skin, subcutaneous fat, the nasal su-perficial musculoaponeurotic system (SMAS), a loose areolar layer that includes deep fatty tissue, followed by perichondrium and periosteum which are bound to the underlying cartilage and bone, respectively. The skin of the upper and middle thirds of the nose is thin and pliable, while the skin overlying the tip is thicker and more fixed to the cartilage framework. The blood supply to the nose arises from both the internal and

external carotid artery systems with contributions predominantly from the terminal branches of the ophthalmic and facial arteries. Named vessels run primarily within and above the nasal-SMAS. Primary arteries are typically paired and run in paramedian and lateral trajectories, and include the dorsal nasal arteries, the external branches of the anterior ethmoid arteries, the lateral nasal arteries, and paired columellar arteries (**Fig. 1**). Each of these has an intricate anastomosis with the others. The arteries each course with corre-sponding veins that are notable for their lack of valves. Venous drainage is provided primarily by the ophthalmic and angular veins. It should be noted, however, that dissections and intraopera-tive observation do occasionally find a dominant midline vessel–especially in the dorsum or colu-mella. Thus, simply keeping injections directly in the midline do not preclude the potential for intra-vascular injection.

CHOICE OF FILLER

Dermal fillers in the United States are classified as temporary or semipermanent. Temporary filler mo-lecular compounds include the aforementioned hyaluronic acids (HA) which are typically members of the JUVÉDERM® (Allergan Aesthetics, Irvine, CA) or *Restylane*® (Galderma, Fort Worth, TX) family of products and calcium hydroxylapatite (CaHA) by RADIESSE® (MERZ North America, Franksville, WI.). Semipermanent polymethylme-thacrylate (PMMA) Bellafill® (Suneva Medical, San Diego, CA) is also used in some practices. Injectable silicone has been used historically, but due to its irreversibility and association with poten-tial migration and/or granuloma formation, its use has largely fallen out of favor.

Fillers are typically classified based on their elasticity and viscosity. Elasticity, or G-prime (G′), explains the degree of filler shape retention when acted upon by an applied external force. In this case, higher the G′, the firmer the substance and less susceptible to deformation. These products tend to provide greater tissue lifting ability. Fillers with lower G′ values are more malleable, disten-sible, and tend to contour more smoothly to the surrounding tissue. Compounds with a high G′ such as *Restylane*® are ideal for the dorsum as they have greater structural integrity, are firm, maintain shape after treatment, and help to lift the overlying tissue.[9] Conversely, low G′ fillers like JUVÉDERM® are ideal for use in the tip and ala as they can be molded to obtain the desired contour.[9] Thus filler choice is dependent not only on physician comfort, preference, and experience but also on the targeted area for application.

INJECTION TECHNIQUE

Several varied techniques have been described for nasal filler injections. These can be divided into top-down and bottom-up approaches and include both needle and cannula injection techniques. In the senior author's experience, injections have overwhelmingly been used more for the upper third and mid-vault of the nose. Therefore, we generally use a top-down approach for injection and use needles for most injections. Cannulas, however, have been used as well, especially in the columella or when injections are placed in a more lateral orientation along the nasal sidewalls or in the trajectory of the lower lateral crura. Cannula use is not a fail-safe, though, against intravascular injection. Their use should not provide a false sense of security against vascular occlusion.

After informed consent and photos are obtained, patients are seated in a semirecumbent position for injections. The chair is limited to only $10°–20°$ of recline, though, to maintain patient comfort, while simultaneously keeping the nose as close to its upright orientation as possible. Injection of anesthetics is avoided to prevent the distortion of the thin, delicate soft tissue envelope and ensure the precision of filler placement and effect. Topical anesthetics can be applied, but have generally been found to be unnecessary. Makeup, if present, is removed and the skin is cleansed with both alcohol and chlorhexidine gluconate 4% antiseptic soap (Hibiclens®, Mölnlycke Health Care Norcross, Georgia). The nondominant thumb and forefinger are used to place bilateral, paramedian compression on the nose in an effort to compress nearby vascular structures while simultaneously slightly tenting the soft tissue envelope upward. A needle is most often used for injection and aimed perpendicular to the skin surface, placing filler in small aliquots deeply in a supraperiosteal/supraperichondrial plane that is below the nasal-SMAS. Volume for each injection is limited to droplets of 0.05 to 0.1 mL per injection site. Aspiration is performed before each injection and the skin is closely observed for any blanching. As material is deposited, it can be shaped if necessary to match the desired nasal contour. Typically, only a portion of the syringe volume is used to obtain the desired result for the entire nose. We err in favor of under injection with plans for patients to observe their results for 7 to 14 days and return for a touchup procedure if needed once the swelling resolves. Postinjection, patients are instructed to resume normal skincare and to use ice for swelling if needed, but to avoid massage and excessive manipulation of the nose and injection sites.

RISKS AND COMPLICATIONS

Filler injections, like any procedure, are associated with risks and complications irrespective of the patient and surgeon involved. And some of these can be particularly devastating. For these reasons, we stress the need for surgeon training and knowledge, facility with filler injections in general, and patient education.

More common risks of injection include redness and mild edema, tenderness, and even bruising at the injection sites. Though rare, infection is also a possibility. Like many areas of the face, superficial injections can produce a bluish hue, or Tyndall effect, which, like intravascular injection, can be avoided by depositing filler below the nasal SMAS. The most serious complications include skin necrosis and injection-related blindness due to vascular occlusion or emboli formation. Skin necrosis can result from either intraarterial injection, which leads to emboli in the terminal vessels, or from filler-induced external compression on the vessels. Blindness results from intraarterial injection under high pressure which causes retrograde arterial embolism to the ophthalmic and retinal arteries. Treatment of skin necrosis consists of nitro paste, aspirin, and injection of hyaluronidase into the field within 4 hours. Treatment of injection-related blindness includes retrobulbar hyaluronidase injection, which must be conducted within 60 to 90 minutes to avoid permanent vision loss. Management for all of these complications is obviously time-sensitive and requires rapid recognition. The surgeon must have immediate access to hyaluronidase and nitroglycerin paste, and ideally, should keep an emergent filler complication kit on hand in the clinic. The patient should also be given aspirin at the time serious complications are noticed. Management of filler complications is discussed elsewhere.[11,12]

PATIENT SELECTION AND APPLICATIONS

There are myriad reasons a patient may opt to proceed with a nonsurgical rhinoplasty as opposed to surgical intervention. Some patients may not have the means available to afford the cost of surgery, while others may want limited recovery time with a more instantaneous result. Additionally, because nonsurgical rhinoplasty is temporary and reversible, patients have the option of seeing first what a surgical rhinoplasty may offer them without the permanence of a surgical procedure. Patients who have previously undergone a surgical rhinoplasty or have some other acquired or congenital nasal deformity may have small contour irregularities that are more easily amenable to filler

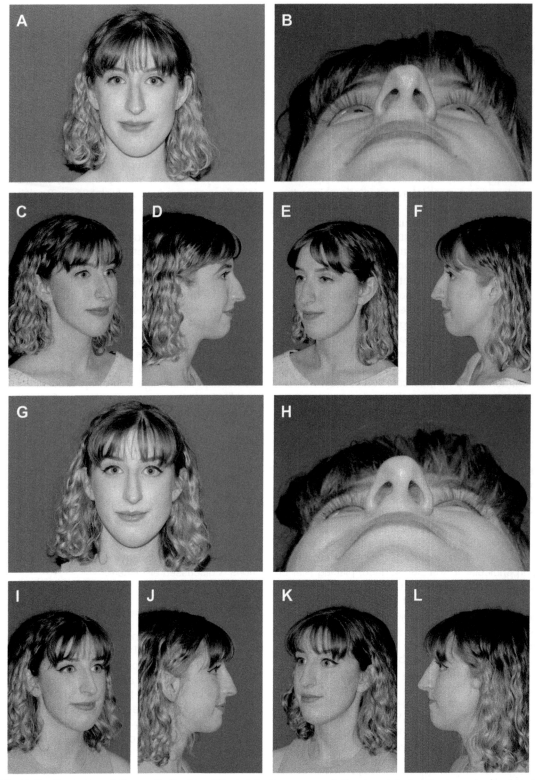

Fig. 2. Profileplasty and the aesthetic dorsal lines. Injection augmentation to minimize the impact of a dorsal hump, improve tip rotation, support, and definition, and correct a right-sided midvault hollow for an improved brow-tip aesthetic line. (*A–F*) – Preinjection. (*G–L*) – Two-weeks postinjection.

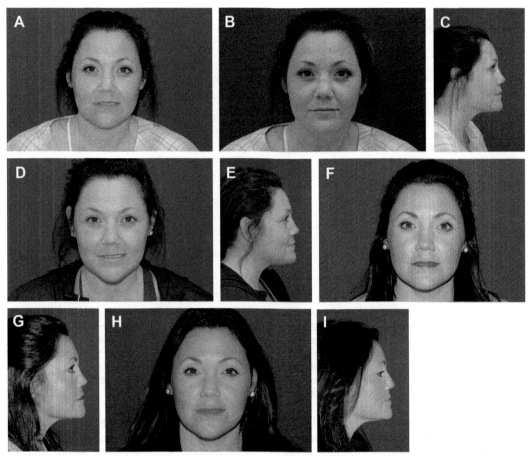

Fig. 3. Acquired nasal deformities. Patient with Wegener's granulomatosis, inverted-V deformity, and early saddle nasal deformity. Filler augmentation was used to efface her midvault and dorsal volume loss. (*A–C*)- Preinjection. Note Fig. 3B use of no-flash photography to help accentuate her topographic discrepancies and shadowing. (*D, E*) – Two-weeks postinjection. (*F, G*) - Twenty-months postinjection demonstrates volume loss from filler resorption. (*H, I*) – Two weeks following touch-up injections at 20-months.

augmentation, as well. And finally, some patients are known to be poor surgical candidates for any number of reasons, leaving in-office injections a viable option.

Because of the growing popularity of liquid rhinoplasty and its presentation in social media formats, patients are increasingly inquiring about this option. Even so, many remain misinformed about the capabilities, limits, and risks of injection augmentation of the nose. These factors seem to be geographically dependent as our personal polling of surgeons has found colleagues with similar observations to ours, while others have seen waning interest in their communities. In any case, it is imperative to educate patients about the fillers themselves, the techniques used, and the fact that this procedure can only *add* volume to the nasal shape and not reduce size or structure in any way. And even though results are more immediate than a surgical procedure, we advocate

photography and pre/postprocedural comparisons in some delayed fashion as the immediate swelling that ensues with injection can cloud the ultimate outcome.

Here, we share several case examples that are representative of liquid rhinoplasty in our practice.

Profileplasty and the Aesthetic Dorsal Lines

One of the more common reasons for patients to seek rhinoplasty is to address a dorsal hump or convexity and improve their profile (**Fig. 2**). This is no different for liquid rhinoplasty. In this case, a young woman presented with an interest in improvement to her profile. Though she was an ideal candidate for surgical rhinoplasty, she was also a professional vocalist who had concerns about maintaining her vocal quality and resonance. As a result, she presented to her consultation having already decided against surgery. To

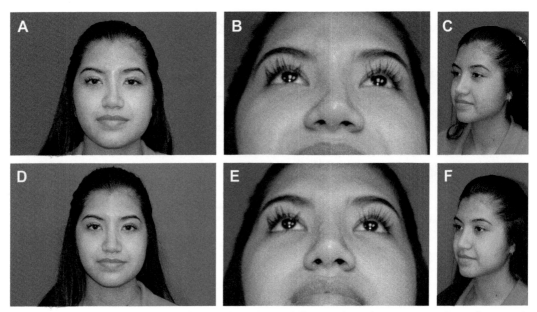

Fig. 4. Postrhinoplasty deformities. In the months and years following rhinoplasty surgery, volume discrepancies and shadowing can become more evident with time. Here, filler augmentation was used instead of revision surgery to help correct a single concern of right mid-vault depression. (*A–C*) – Preinjection. 18-month postoperative views with evidence of right midvault hollowing. This is evident in the anterior base and three-quarters views. There were no dorsal concerns on the profile. (*D–F*)- Postinjection. Immediately following injection there is improved midvault symmetry. There is marked early swelling as well, though, which should be reassessed in the weeks following injection to ensure the restoration of the desired volume.

help achieve her desired result, the radix and supratip were first augmented. Next, tip support was added through a columellar injection to help with a slight increase in rotation. The rhinoplasty surgeon is well aware of intraoperative local anesthetic injections which tend to demonstrate how the addition of volume increases turgor pressure, especially in the tip complex. The on-table result can be an immediate increase in tip support, rotation, and projection. Here, a cannula was used to augment the columella much like a columellar strut, stiffening the tip complex, and increasing a few degrees of rotation. This also helped efface an interarticular depression that alluded to bifidity in the infratip. Finally, the right mid-vault concavity was also addressed to create a smoother brow-tip aesthetic line.

Acquired Nasal Deformities

Some patients are not ideal rhinoplasty candidates. In this case, a middle-aged woman was referred by our laryngology colleagues for the evaluation of perceived nasal shadowing, mid-vault collapse, and an early dorsal saddle (**Fig. 3**). She was a patient with dysphonia that had recently been diagnosed with Wegener's granulomatosis. Fortunately, she had no septal perforation and her endonasal examination was completely

normal. As her disease, though, was recently diagnosed and future progression uncertain, nonsurgical options were explored along with our traditional discussions of surgical rhinoplasty. Filler augmentation was ultimately decided on, and in this case, helped to ameliorate an inverted-V deformity and create a smoother nasal profile. She has now been followed for several years. Volume was found to show a noticeable decrease at 20-month, at which time additional HA was added.

Postrhinoplasty Deformities

As swelling resolves and the soft tissue envelope contracts, skeletal and cartilage discrepancies can become more evident after rhinoplasty (**Figs. 4** and **5**). Depending on the timing after surgery, the patient's interest in revision surgery, and risk of surgery compared with the benefit sought by surgeon and patient, filler augmentation may be a viable adjunct to correct aesthetic discrepancies. Similar to the cases above, this first case (see **Fig. 4**) involved the correction of a mid-vault concavity without any profile concerns. This improved her middle third width and symmetry, thereby eliminating undesirable shadowing and improving her brow-tip aesthetic line.

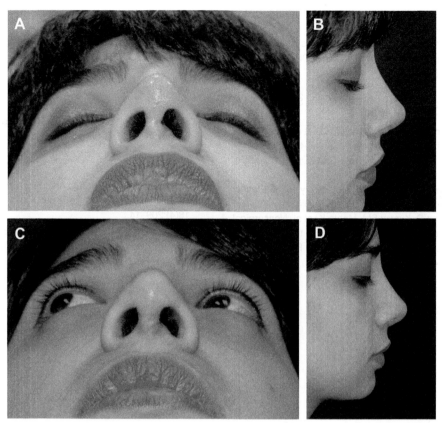

Fig. 5. Postrhinoplasty deformities. Following open rhinoplasty with another surgeon, this patient presented with dissatisfaction with her columella. She was particularly unhappy with her profile in photos. As her wedding was approaching, formal surgical correction was felt to be contraindicated in the short term. Therefore, scar revision and filler augmentation were used to correct the columellar discrepancies. (*A, B*)- Preinjection. (*C, D*)- Postinjection and scar revision.

In the second case (**Fig. 5**), a patient presented having undergone rhinoplasty with another surgeon. She was unhappy with her columella and infratip after healing from a stair-step incision used in an open approach surgery. She, too, was a revision surgery candidate, but presented within a few months of her upcoming wedding. Here, a limited scar revision was performed followed by volume augmentation to correct soft tissue and cartilage deformities in the columella. This improved not only her base view but the infratip was also smoother in profile.

SUMMARY

The popularity of "liquid", or nonsurgical, rhinoplasty has grown considerably over the last decade. While some practices have seen a plateau or decrease in patient requests for liquid rhinoplasty, many continue to see a rise that coincides with the increase in visibility on social media. Though attractive to both patient and surgeon for a multitude of reasons, nasal filler injections are not without risk. Patient education, knowledge of nasal surgical anatomy, and understanding of the management of complications are critical for safe, viable incorporation of liquid rhinoplasty into the surgeon's practice.

REFERENCES

1. Plastic surgery Statistics report. American Society of Plastic Surgeons. Available at: https://www.plasticsurgery.org/documents/News/Statistics/2020/plastic-surgery-statistics-full-report-2020.pdf. Accessed October 18, 2021.
2. Plastic surgery Statistics report. American Society of Plastic Surgeons. Available at: https://www.plasticsurgery.org/documents/News/Statistics/2019/plastic-surgery-statistics-full-report-20219.pdf. Accessed October 18, 2021.
3. Plastic surgery Statistics report. American Society of Plastic Surgeons. Available at: https://www.plasticsurgery.org/documents/News/Statistics/2010/

plastic-surgery-statistics-full-report-2010.pdf. Accessed October 18, 2021.

4. Beer KR. Nasal reconstruction using 20 mg/ml cross-linked hyaluronic acid. J Drugs Dermatol 2006;5(5):465–6.

5. Mehta U, Fridirici Z. Advanced techniques in nonsurgical rhinoplasty. Facial Plast Surg Clin North Am 2019;27(3):355–65.

6. Rohrich RJ, Agrawal N, Avashia Y, et al. Safety in the use of fillers in nasal augmentation—the liquid rhinoplasty. Plast Reconstr Surg Glob Open 2020;8(8): e2820.

7. Raggio BS, Asaria J. Filler rhinoplasty. In: StatPearls. Treasure Island (FL): StatPearls Publishing; 2021.

8. Williams LC, Kidwai SM, Mehta K, et al. Nonsurgical rhinoplasty: a systematic review of technique, outcomes, and complications. Plast Reconstr Surg 2020;146(1):41–51.

9. Kurkjian T, Jonathan MD, Ahmad J, Rohrich RJ. Soft-tissue fillers in rhinoplasty. Plast Reconstr Surg 2014; 133(2):121e–6e.

10. Redaelli A. Medical rhinoplasty with hyaluronic acid and botulinum toxin a: a very simple and quite effective technique. J Cosmet Dermatol 2008;7(3): 210–20.

11. Johnson ON 3rd, Kontis TC. Nonsurgical rhinoplasty. Facial Plast Surg 2016;32(5):500–6.

12. Patel RG. Nasal anatomy and function. Facial Plast Surg 2017;33(1):3–8.

13. Lam SM, Williams EF 3rd. Anatomic considerations in aesthetic rhinoplasty. Facial Plast Surg 2002; 18(4):209–14.

14. Kontis TC, Bunin L, Fitzgerald R. Injectable fillers: panel discussion, controversies, and techniques. Facial Plast Surg Clin North Am 2018;26(2):225–36.

Creating Ideal Lips with Toxins and Fillers

Myriam Loyo, MD, MCR[a],*, Theda Kontis, MD[b]

KEYWORDS

- Lip augmentation • Hyaluronic acid fillers • Neurotoxin

KEY POINTS

- When comparing the volume of the upper to lower lip, traditionally a 2:3 ratio was desirable for Caucasian women and 1:1 for women of color. Increasingly a ratio of 1:1 is sought in all races.
- The labial arteries are most commonly located submucosally but can also be present in the muscle or subcutaneously.
- Avoid overfilling by appreciating the subunits and natural contour of the lip.
- Swelling and bruising are the most common complication after lip augmentation. Herpes simplex virus (HSV-1) eruptions, vascular occlusion, product migration, nodule formation, and infection can occur after lip augmentation.

INTRODUCTION

The lips are a central and essential feature of facial appearance and esthetics. When looking at attractive faces, we spent most of our time observing the eyes and lips although the rest of the facial features fade away.[1] Full lips are beautiful and youthful.[2] Treatments to enhance the lips have long been pursued. Silicone injections were popular in the 1960s and collagen injections in the 1970s. Also, during the 1970s surgical lip implants with expanded polytetrafluororethylene (Gortex®) were widely used a longer-lasting alternative to collagen injections.[3] In the 1990s, hyaluronic acid fillers (HA fillers) revolutionized the market for facial esthetics. HA fillers' safety profile, quick recovery, and natural results have made it the preferred option for lip enhancement with or without complementary neurotoxin. Not surprisingly, lip enhancement has gained widespread, immense popularity.

In this article, we will discuss how to evaluate and treat the lip with HA filler and neurotoxin. We will discuss desired esthetic of the natural and attractive lips and how "influencers" and social media are changing our goals with lip augmentation. The expected changes of the lip with aging will be reviewed. Descriptions of how to treat the lips and diagrams and before and after photos will be included. Finally, we will discuss how to manage complications of treatment including a case study of late-onset nodule formation.

DISCUSSION

Evaluation and Goals

Most patients who present for lip rejuvenation are looking for enhancement by augmenting the lips. Recognizing is no universal ideal standard for beautiful lips, we will discuss concepts that apply to beauty in the lips that may aid in achieving the best results possible. Fullness of the lips, curved

Conflict of interest: Dr T. Kontis is an Allergan and Galderma investigator and Bureau speaker. Dr M. Loyo has no conflicts of interest.
[a] Division of Facial Plastic & Reconstructive Surgery, Department of Otolaryngology & Head and Neck Surgery, Oregon Health & Sciences University, CH5E, 3303 SW Bond Avenue, Portland, OR 97239, USA; [b] Department of Otolaryngology-Head and Neck Surgery, Department of Plastic and Reconstructive Surgery, Johns Hopkins, 1838 Greene Tree Road, Suite 370, Baltimore, MD 21208, USA
* Corresponding author.
E-mail address: loyo@ohsu.edu

Cupid's bow, and strong definition of the philtrum are considered beautiful and youthful; loss of lip fullness, thinning of the vermilion, and flattening of the lips are less desirable and associated with aging. Younger patients may seek beauty enhancement although older patients might also be looking to correct aging.

Evaluating the lips requires evaluating the entire anatomic area in the context of the face. Traditionally, it has been considered natural to have a slightly smaller upper lip compared with the lower lip. A ratio of 2:3 has been recommended for Caucasians, whereas in women of color it approaches 1:1. More recently, as fuller lips have become more acceptable, a ratio of 1:1 has gained popularity in all races.[4] Additionally, the upper lip should project forward slightly more than the lower. The following measurements have been described to evaluate lip projection on profile. Drawing a straight line from subnasal to the soft tissue pogonion and a perpendicular line to the most anterior portion of the lip, the upper lip should lie 3.5 mm anterior to that line and the lower lip 2.2 mm. If a straight line is drawn from the nasal tip to the pogonion. The upper lip should lie 4 mm behind the line and the lower lip 2 mm behind it.[5] The anatomic facial subunits of the lips extend from the base of the nose superiorly to the chin inferiorly and are limited laterally by the nasolabial folds and labiomental folds. Evaluating these areas is particularly important when our goal is facial rejuvenation. Vertical rhytids in the cutaneous upper lip, lengthening of the cutaneous upper lip, depression of the oral commissures, and deep labiomental grooves are signs of aging. It is important to remember skeletal and dental support also affects the position of the lips.

Discussing with our patients their specific goals and desired changes is key in achieving patient satisfaction. Although most patients are looking to add natural fullness to the lips, it is helpful to discuss which specific areas of the lips they would like to concentrate on. Some patients seek volume evenly throughout the lips while other want to concentrate in a specific area. A common request is the vertical lengthening of the upper lip in the front view. Inquire about fine lines on the lips, the vermilion border, or on the cutaneous lip. Discuss any asymmetries, scars, or nevi in the lips. Evaluating the lips at rest and during smile can help evaluate dental and gum show during smile to plan treatment. Rarely, will a patient describe the philtrum as a primary complaint. As providers, we can explain how enhancing the philtrum can improve definition in Cupid's bow and add projection to the upper lip.

As we plan our treatment, understanding the lip vasculature is important to avoid vascular complications with filler injection. The layers of the red lip include the epidermis, subcutaneous tissue, orbicularis oris muscle fibers, and mucosa. The labial arteries are typically located posterior to the free edge of the lip, submucosally between the mucosa and the orbicularis oris muscle. Importantly, many studies have shown although the labial arteries are most commonly submucosally (>70% of cases), they can also be located intramuscularly or subcutaneously.[6–8] The vermiliocutaneous junction is marked by the white roll. HA filler is typically injected anterior to the muscle along the surface of the lip and along the vermilion border. Precision is important in this area as the depth from the surface of the vermilion border to the superior labial artery is less than 4 mm.[9,10]

Current Evidence

At the time we are writing this review, six HA fillers have been approved by the Food and Drug Administration (FDA) for their use in lip augmentation. The major categories are Juvéderm and Restylane (**Table 1**). Juvéderm is manufactured by Allergan by crosslinking nonanimal stabilized hyaluronic acid (NASHA) to 1,4-butanediol diglyceryl ether (BDDE). Juvéderm products are monophasic gels. The original products are produced by Hylacross technology, which allows Juvéderm Ultra to have 9% crosslinking.[11] More recent Juvéderm products use Vycross technology and combine HA of different weight. Volbella combines low molecular weight HA with a high degree of crosslinking and has a final concentration of 15 mg/mL.[12] Restylane is manufactured by Galderma Laboratories and is also a BDDE-crosslinked NASHA product. Restylane products are biphasic gels with particulate sizes ranging from 330 to 430 μm. Their degree of crosslinking is relatively low at 1%, and their concentration is 20 mg/mL.[13] Restylane silk was the first filler to be approved by the FDA for lip augmentation. The newer generation Restylane products are manufactured with XpresHAn Technology, which allows for varying degrees of crosslinking. The most recent filler to be approved by the FDA for lip augmentation was Retylane Kysse in 2020. Restylane Kysse has 7% crosslinking, which is higher than Restylane Refyne (6%) but lower than Restylane Defyne (8%).[14] A 2018 randomized, blinded trial comparing Restylane Kysse to Juvéderm Volbella sponsored by Galderma Laboratories revealed similar satisfaction and durability of the products, with slightly less volume needed for Restylane Kysse to achieve the desired results. The mean volume needed to improve 1 grade in the Lip Fullness Grading Scale was 1.54 mL with

Table 1
Hyaluronic acid (HA) fillers approved by the Food and Drug Administration (FDA) for lip augmentation

Product (Manufacturer)	Approval Date	Material	G'[19]	Crosslinking Technology (%)	References
Juvéderm Ultra XC (HYC-24) (Allergan, Inc)	2015	24 mg/mL HA, lidocaine 0.3%	207	Hylacross (9%)	Dayan et al,[20] 2015 and Bogdan Allemann and Baumann[11] 2008
Juvéderm Volbella XC (VYC-15L) (Allergan, Inc)	2016	15 mg/mL HA, lidocaine 0.3%	274	Vycross (NA)	Raspaldo et al,[21] 2015
Restylane (Galderman Laboratories, LP)	2011	20 mg/mL HA	544	NASHA (1%)	Glogau et al.[22] 2012 and Solish and Swift[23] 2011
Restylane- L (Galderman Laboratories, LP)	2012	20 mg/mL HA, lidocaine 0.3%	544	NASHA (1%)	Raspaldo et al,[21] 2015
Restylane silk (Galderman Laboratories, LP)	2014	20 mg/mL HA, lidocaine 0.3%	344	NASHA (1%)	Chiu et al,[24] 2016
Restylane Kysse (Galderman Laboratories, LP)	2020	20 mg/mL HA, lidocaine 0.3%	151	XpresHAn (7%)	Hilton et al.[15] 2018

Abbreviation: NASHA, nonanimal stabilized hyaluronic acid.

Restylane Kysse (standard deviation [SD] 0.36) versus 1.94 mL with Juvéderm Volbella (SD 0.34)[15] Although only six products have a specific indication for lip augmentation, several other HA facial fillers are available in the United States. Belotero Balance from Merz Aesthetics and Resilient Hyaluronic Acid (RHA) 2, 3, and 4 from Teoxane are also HA fillers available in the United States, but they are much less commonly used and not currently indicated for lip augmentation by the FDA. Hyamax Kiss and Emervel Lips are both used for lip augmentation abroad but not available in the United States.[16,17] The different characteristics of the HA fillers determine their expected result including their cohesivity, elasticity, and duration. Higher concentration and higher crosslinking give products more stiffness and increase their duration; they also make them more resistant to hyaluronidase. In general, HA fillers of the Juvéderm family are more resistant to biodegradation with hyaluronidase than fillers of the Restylane family.[18]

Combining hyaluronic acid filler with botulinum toxin type A has become widely accepted and increasingly popular. The value of combing them for enhanced efficacy has been recognized by several expert panels including the Global Aesthetic Consensus group.[25] Around the lips, botulinum toxin type A can be used to target the orbicularis oris, depressor anguli oris, or mentalis muscles. Treatment to these areas can enhance the lips, soften perioral rhytids, lift the oral commissure, soften labiomental lines, and treat an overactive mentalis (particularly in cases of retrognathia). A 2010, multicenter, randomized, parallel study comparing lower facial rejuvenation with HA filler alone (Juvéderm Ultra or Juvéderm Ultra Plus), onabotulinumtoxin A alone, or a combination of both, found the combination treatment achieved better results in perioral, lip fullness, and oral commissure assessments.[26,27]

Approach/Injection Technique

Appreciation of the lip esthetic subunits[2] is crucial for augmenting the lips into a beautiful appearance rather than just "filling a sausage." Patents are often leery about receiving lip injections because many fear being overfilled. Certainly, some patients want to look overfilled, although others just want to improve, but not over-do, their lip anatomy. It is important to first understand the patient's goals before proceeding with lip injections. In addition, the unique lip anatomy needs to be addressed. Does the patient want definition and/or volume? How much volume do they want? Are their lip proportions appropriate or do they need correction? Are the lips symmetric? Once these questions have been answered, then injector will have a good idea how to proceed with injections to produce a happy patient. It is also important to inform the patient that they will

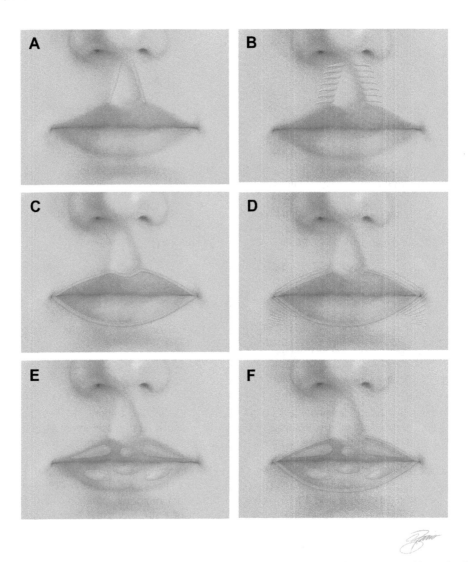

Fig. 1. Diagram showing lip filler injection techniques. (A) Philtral columns can be augmented linearly along the fold. (B) Alternatively, the phitral columns can be augmented with small horizontal retrograde injections injected medial to lateral. (C) Definition of the lips is accomplished by augmenting the vermilion border, injection either retrograde or anterograde, from lateral to medial. (D) Small amount of filler may be placed outside the vermilion border after injection to decrease shadowing. (E) Lip fullness is achieved by direct injection into the body of the lips, artistically filling in deficient areas. (F) A combination of these techniques may be necessary to achieve the desired results. (From Kontis TC and Lacombe V, Cosmetic Injection Techniques, 2nd edition, Thieme Medical Publishers, Inc.)

feel their lips look too big immediately after the injection is finished, and they will need a few days for the swelling and bruising to improve before their final result. Techniques vary depending on the patient's desires and anatomy (Fig. 1). Occasionally patients just want correction of asymmetries. Many "older" women just desire bringing their shriveled lips "back to life." This includes correction of circumoral lines, improving volume loss, defining the philtral columns, or improving the vermillion definition.

Despite HA fillers with lidocaine, injection of filler into the lips is somewhat painful. Some patients can tolerate without anesthesia, but anesthetic treatments can include topical lidocaine/prilocaine (2.5%–2.5%), "dental block" with 1% or 2% lidocaine, and/or augmented with nitrous oxide (Pronox). The patient's lips should be cleaned with alcohol pads before injection, and informed consent obtained. Preinjection photos are recommended. Usually, the patient is in a sitting or semi-recumbent position, and the injector injects laterally to medially, moving from one side of the patient to the other.

Vermillion injection is performed to improve the definition of the vermillion border and Cupid's bow. This is one of the few areas where an anterograde injection is possible. The injector places the needle into the vermillion border and injects without moving the needle and can observe the filler track along the vermillion in the potential space. This technique is nice for the improvement of smoker's lines and to improve definition. It can accentuate lip eversion; however, it does not volumize the lips.

Lip volumization techniques vary by the injector. For volume, the filler can be placed symmetrically in the body of the lip starting at the wet line. Injections also are performed laterally to medially, from each side of the patient. Care must be taken to avoid intravascular injection into the labial artery. It is important to respect appropriate lip esthetic proportions when adding lip volume. Remember the traditional recommendation of the upper lip:lower lip ratio for Caucasians is 2:3, whereas in women of color it approaches 1:1 and the recent trends toward 1:1 for all races.

Perioral treatments also can improve the overall appearance of the lips. The oral commissures, for example, can be elevated by using a filler or by placing a small amount of neurotoxin in the depressor anguli oris muscle. Similarly, the vertical rhytids or "smoker's lines" can be improved by injection of small amounts of filler in the lip lines and can be augmented by a neurotoxin (**Fig. 2**).

Aftercare includes valacyclovir (500 mg/d for 1 week) if the patient has a herpes simplex history as lip injections can trigger a recurrence. Ice is applied by the patient for the first 24 hours to treat expected bruising and swelling. Patients should be counseled that their lips are swollen once they leave the office and will diminish in size somewhat in a few days. Examples of before and after photos of patients treated with lip augmentation by the authors are shown in **Fig. 3**.

The Role of Social Media

Social media and "influencers" had a major impact on the injectables market by both increasing awareness and developing or re-naming techniques that patients request. Some of these "designer" lip injections include the Russian Lip, the Keyhole Lip, and the Lip Flip.

The "Russian Lip" technique is performed by changing the direction of the injection from horizontal to vertical. The needle is inserted at the wet line and tracks submucosally to vertically the vermillion border, where a thread of filler is then placed via retrograde technique. This is then performed in multiple tracks along the lip. The result is a full lip with increased eversion of the vermillion.

The "Keyhole Lip" or "Jolie lip" is performed to create an indentation in the center of the lip. When done in the upper and lower lips, it creates a central "keyhole." This technique was created to emulate the lower lip central crease of Angela Jolie's lower lip. The procedure is performed by taking a piece of dental floss knotted at one end and threading it between the incisors to place the knot behind the incisors. The floss is then pulled tightly into the lip to form an indentation (**Fig. 4**). Although the patient holds the floss tightly, the injector places filler on either side of the lip. Removing the floss then reveals an indentation.

Social media has also served to increase patient awareness of the "lip flip." Experienced injectors have performed this injection technique for many years to improve "smoker's lines." (**Fig. 5**) In some of these patients, release of the downward pull of the orbicularis muscle will elevate the pink lip slightly. This technique involves using 1 to 2 units of onabotulinumtoxin A in each injection placed symmetrically on the vermilion border. This procedure works best in patients who have a strong downward pull of the orbicularis oris muscle. The results are subtle and this procedure appeals to patients who are anxious about having overfilled lips.

Complications

Swelling and bruising

The most common complications of lip injections include swelling and bruising. Patients are asked to discontinue oral anticoagulants like aspirin and nonsteroidal anti-inflammatory drugs and vitamins 10 to 14 days before treatment, if medically advisable. Immediately after injection, ice packs can help with bruising and discomfort. Oral preparations with bromelain and arnica have been found

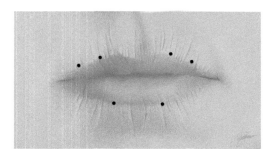

Fig. 2. Diagram showing the injection technique for perioral vertical lines or "smoker lines". (*From* Kontis TC and Lacombe V, Cosmetic Injection Techniques, 2nd edition, Thieme Medical Publishers, Inc.)

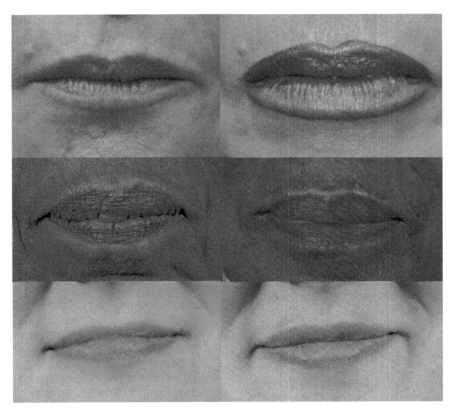

Fig. 3. Before and after photos of patients treated with lip augmentation.

helpful in the reduction of bruising, as well as arnica or Vitamin K gels placed topically on the bruises. It is not uncommon for patients to leave the office complaining their lips are too big, then call a week later saying "it's all gone, I like ed them better when they were swollen!" Therefore, managing patient expectations is important, and taking preinjection photos are crucial in these patients.

Herpes simplex
Herpes simplex virus (HSV-1) eruptions can be triggered by lip injections. All patients with a history of fever blisters should be placed on valacyclovir (500 mg) daily for 5 to 7 days after injection. Patients with active or recent eruptions should delay receiving injections for a few weeks until the lesion has completely healed.

Vascular occlusion
Vascular occlusion of the labial arteries is possible but uncommon. Some injectors feel

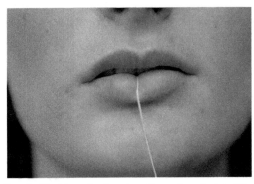

Fig. 4. Photograph showing the setup for a "Key hole" injection of the lower lip.

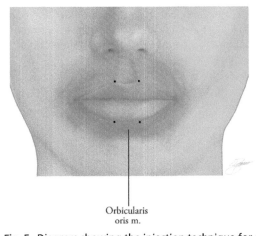

Orbicularis
oris m.

Fig. 5. Diagram showing the injection technique for a "Lip Flip". (*From* Kontis TC and Lacombe V, Cosmetic Injection Techniques, 2nd edition, Thieme Medical Publishers, Inc.)

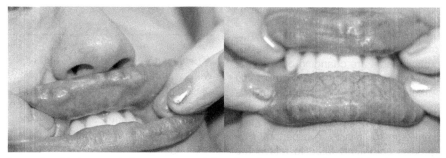

Fig. 6. Photographs of late-onset inflammatory nodules after lip augmentation with hyaluronic acid fillers.

cannula use guarantees safety, but others feel precise contouring is not possible without needle use. The labial arteries are located most commonly in the submocusal or intramuscular region; therefore superficial injection planes should be followed for filler injection.[7] If the lip blanches during injection, the injection should stop and the area massaged and warm compresses placed. If the area does not respond to these initial treatments, protocols for the management of intravascular injection should be followed. These include injection with hyaluronidase, oral aspirin, nitropaste application, and close follow-up.

Product migration

Product migration can occur in the lips, often because of the continuous effects of motion on the filler. These early appearing effects and nodules (less than 1 month) are usually considered to be common and resolve over time, usually without intervention.[28] The filler may migrate within the confines of the lip to produce a palpable lump, may migrate close to the lip surface producing a bluish hue, or may migrate outside the confines of the pink lip. For asymmetric lumps on the lip, after waiting 2 weeks for bruising and swelling to resolve, these lumps can occasionally be massaged or compressed. However, bluish appearing nodules (Tyndall effect), likely require treatment with either hyaluronidase or direct exproosion of the product. The lumps can quickly be reduced by use of a 20 G needle inserted directly into the lump, and the product is expressed by gentle pressure. Asymmetries outside the confines of the pink lip into the lip skin may require small amounts of hyaluronidase for improved contouring.

Nodules

Delayed-onset nodules (greater than 1 month) suggest and inflammatory or infectious process, especially when the nodules are inflamed and tender. The role of biofilms in these cases has received particular attention in the recent years.[29]

Treatment of late-onset inflammatory nodules can include oral steroids, antibiotics (doxycycline or minocycline), and intralesional injection of triamcinolone, 5-fluorouracil, and/or hyaluronidase.[30]

Infection

Infection is an uncommon complication after filler injection, provided that the area was cleaned well before injection, and the proper technique is used. If a severe infection is noted after filler injection, the abscess should be drained and the purulent material sent for culture/sensitivity. Treatment should include a macrolide and quinolone antibiotic for 10–14 days.

Alternative Treatments

This review concentrated on the use of HA filler and neurotoxin to enhance the lips. However, it is possible to reshape the lips with surgical interventions. Typically, patients seeking surgical intervention are looking for longer-lasting results than HA fillers, and neurotoxin can provide. In certain instances, surgical procedures can provide results that are not possible with nonsurgical techniques. For example, the subnasal lip lift can be used to shorten an overly long cutaneous upper lip although also improving red lip show.[31–33] Lip advancements at the commissure or vermilion border can also be used to enhance the lips.[34] Lip augmentation with fat grafting, autologous soft tissue, or polytetrafluoroethylene grafts is also possible.[35,36] Incisions in the lips carry the risks of scarring; augmentation with fat has the risk of unpredictable reabsorption, pressure necrosis, and vascular occlusion.

In cases where skin texture and vertical rhytids of the upper lip are the main concern, laser resurfacing can be a powerful treatment to use sequentially with HA filler and neurotoxin to achieve the desired lip outcomes.[37] Dermabrasion, chemical peels, and other nonsurgical skin rejuvenation techniques have also been shown to be effective in this area.[34,38] A separate review in this editorial discusses skin rejuvenation.

SUMMARY

Lip enhancement with HA filler and neurotoxin has gained widespread popularity. Influencers, celebrities, and social media are changing our cultural normal and esthetic perception making fuller lips more acceptable and desirable. Treatments that enhance lip volume and shape and rejuvenates the perioral region are widely sought after. Lifting the oral commissures and softening perioral rhytids are strategies commonly used to rejuvenate the perioral rejuvenation. Treatment to the lip and perioral region leads to high satisfaction and has relatively low rates of adverse reactions. Combination treatments of HA fillers and neurotoxin have improved results than either treatment by itself. Clinicians offering lip enhancement should prepare to treat complications of lip augmentation such as herpes simplex reactivation, nodule formation, and vascular occlusion.

CLINICS CARE POINTS

1) When comparing the volume of the upper to lower lip, traditionally a 2:3 ratio was desirable for Caucasian women and 1:1 for women of color. Increasingly a ratio of 1:1 is sought in all races.

2) The labial arteries are most commonly located submucosally but can also be present in the muscle or subcutaneously.

3) Six HA fillers are currently approved by the FDA for lip augmentation: Restylane, Restylane-L, Restylane silk, Restylane Kysse, Juvéderm Ultra, and Juvéderm Volbella

4) Patients treated with HA filler for lip augmentation have high satisfaction rates and relatively low complications

5) Avoid overfilling by appreciating the subunits and natural contour of the lip

6) Neurotoxin can be used to treat the depressor anguli oris muscle and lift the corner of the mouth

7) Neurotoxin can be used to treat the orbicularis oris muscle to achieve a "Lip Flip"

8) Swelling and bruising are the most common complications after lip augmentation

9) HSV-1 eruptions can be triggered by lip injections and patients with a history of herpes simplex in the lips should be placed on prophylactic antivirals

10) Vascular occlusion, product migration, nodule formation, and infection can occur after lip augmentation

CASE STUDY
Late-Onset Inflammatory Nodules

Presentation
A healthy 45-year-old female esthetician presents with painful lip nodules. She had 1 cc of HA filler placed in her lips 4 months ago by a certified nurse injector. She was pleased with the cosmetic results until 1 month ago when she developed severely swollen and tender lips, worse in the morning. She returned to her injector, who placed her on a methylprednisolone dose pack and injected the nodules with hyaluronidase. In follow-up, the patient did not respond to the steroid dose pack, so she was placed on high-dose oral prednisone and received two subsequent hyaluronidase injections.

She presented as shown in **Fig. 6**. Examination revealed multiple, extremely tender, firm nodules of the upper and lower lips. She was taking clindamycin for some recent dental work (which occurred after the nodules formed). She had a history of HSV-1 and was also taking valacyclovir.

How would you treat this patient?
The nodules were injected with Kenalog/5-fluorouracil. At 2 weeks, most of the nodules were gone. The few remaining nodules were similarly injected. At her 2-week follow-up visit, all nodules were completely resolved.

DISCUSSION

Nodules forming after hyaluronic acid injection are classified as early (<1 month), or late onset (>1 month), and as either inflammatory or noninflammatory. In this patient case, the nodules were late-onset inflammatory nodules. Early nodules that are noninflammatory (firm but nontender) are generally due to improper placement or product migration. These can be managed expectantly or with massage/product expression or hyaluronidase. Early-onset inflammatory nodules are painful and erythematous, denoting a likely infectious process. Treatment should be performed immediately with oral macrolide and quinolone and possibly incision and drainage with culture.

Some of the longer lasting, more cross-linked hyaluronic acids (Vycross technology) have been associated with late-onset nodules. Delayed-onset nodules are most likely immune response mediated. The first line of treatment would include oral steroids. Hyaluronidase injections are also considered, but fillers with Vycross technology often require higher amounts of hyaluronidase. Nodules that are resistant to this treatment can be injected with triamcinolone with or without the addition of 5-fluorouracil.[30]

REFERENCES

1. Godoy A, et al. The straight truth: measuring observer attention to the crooked nose. Laryngoscope 2011;121(5):937–41.
2. Jacono AA. A new classification of lip zones to customize injectable lip augmentation. Arch Facial Plast Surg 2008;10(1):25–9.
3. Sarnoff DS, Saini R, Gotkin RH. Comparison of filling agents for lip augmentation. Aesthet Surg J 2008; 28(5):556–63.
4. Heidekrueger PI, et al. The current preferred female lip ratio. J Craniomaxillofac Surg 2017;45(5):655–60.
5. Papel ID. Facial plastic and reconstructive surgery. 4th edition. Thieme; 2016.
6. Tansatit T, Apinuntrum P, Phetudom T. A typical pattern of the labial arteries with implication for lip augmentation with injectable fillers. Aesthetic Plast Surg 2014;38(6):1083–9.
7. Cotofana S, et al. Distribution pattern of the superior and inferior labial arteries: impact for safe upper and lower lip augmentation procedures. Plast Reconstr Surg 2017;139(5):1075–82.
8. Pinar YA, Bilge O, Govsa F. Anatomic study of the blood supply of perioral region. Clin Anat 2005; 18(5):330–9.
9. Magden O, et al. Cadaveric study of the arterial anatomy of the upper lip. Plast Reconstr Surg 2004;114(2):355–9.
10. Edizer M, et al. Arterial anatomy of the lower lip: a cadaveric study. Plast Reconstr Surg 2003;111(7): 2176–81.
11. Bogdan Allemann I, Baumann L. Hyaluronic acid gel (Juvederm) preparations in the treatment of facial wrinkles and folds. Clin Interv Aging 2008;3(4): 629–34.
12. Raspaldo H, et al. Juvederm volbella with lidocaine for lip and perioral enhancement: a prospective, randomized, controlled trial. Plast Reconstr Surg Glob Open 2015;3(3):e321.
13. Monheit GD, et al. Novel hyaluronic acid dermal filler: dermal gel extra physical properties and clinical outcomes. Dermatol Surg 2010;36(Suppl 3): 1833–41.
14. Philipp-Dormston WG, et al. Evaluating perceived naturalness of facial expression after fillers to the nasolabial folds and lower face with standardized video and photography. Dermatol Surg 2018;44(6): 826–32.
15. Hilton S, et al. Randomized, evaluator-blinded study comparing safety and effect of two hyaluronic acid gels for lips enhancement. Dermatol Surg 2018; 44(2):261–9.
16. Yazdanparast T, et al. Assessment of the efficacy and safety of hyaluronic acid gel injection in the restoration of fullness of the upper lips. J Cutan Aesthet Surg 2017;10(2):101–5.
17. Farhi D, et al. The Emervel French survey: a prospective real-practice descriptive study of 1,822 patients treated for facial rejuvenation with a new hyaluronic acid filler. J Drugs Dermatol 2013;12(5): e88–93.
18. RZ PMS. The interaction between hyaluronidase and hyaluronic acid gel fillers - a review of the literature and comparative analysis. Plast Aesthet Res 2020; 7(36).
19. Rohrich RJ, Bartlett EL, Dayan E. Practical approach and safety of hyaluronic acid fillers. Plast Reconstr Surg Glob Open 2019;7(6):e2172.
20. Dayan S, et al. Safety and effectiveness of the hyaluronic acid filler, HYC-24L, for lip and perioral augmentation. Dermatol Surg 2015;41(Suppl 1): S293–301.
21. Raspaldo H, et al. Lip and perioral enhancement: a 12-month prospective, randomized, controlled study. J Drugs Dermatol 2015;14(12):1444–52.
22. Glogau RG, et al. A randomized, evaluator-blinded, controlled study of the effectiveness and safety of small gel particle hyaluronic acid for lip augmentation. Dermatol Surg 2012;38(7 Pt 2): 1180–92.
23. Solish N, Swift A. An open-label, pilot study to assess the effectiveness and safety of hyaluronic acid gel in the restoration of soft tissue fullness of the lips. J Drugs Dermatol 2011;10(2):145–9.
24. Chiu A, et al. Lip injection techniques using small-particle hyaluronic acid dermal filler. J Drugs Dermatol 2016;15(9):1076–82.
25. Sundaram H, et al. Global aesthetics consensus: hyaluronic acid fillers and botulinum toxin type A-Recommendations for combined treatment and optimizing outcomes in diverse patient populations. Plast Reconstr Surg 2016;137(5):1410–23.
26. Carruthers A, et al. Multicenter, randomized, parallel-group study of the safety and effectiveness of onabotulinumtoxinA and hyaluronic acid dermal fillers (24-mg/ml smooth, cohesive gel) alone and in combination for lower facial rejuvenation. Dermatol Surg 2010;36(Suppl 4):2121–34.
27. Carruthers J, et al. Multicenter, randomized, parallel-group study of onabotulinumtoxinA and hyaluronic acid dermal fillers (24-mg/ml smooth, cohesive gel) alone and in combination for lower facial rejuvenation: satisfaction and patient-reported outcomes. Dermatol Surg 2010;36(Suppl 4):2135–45.
28. Gupta A, Miller PJ. Management of lip complications. Facial Plast Surg Clin North Am 2019;27(4): 565–70.
29. Safran T, et al. Evaluating safety in hyaluronic acid lip injections. Expert Opin Drug Saf 2021;20(12): 1473–86.
30. Jones DH, et al. Preventing and Treating adverse events of injectable fillers: evidence-based recommendations from the american society for

dermatologic surgery multidisciplinary task force. Dermatol Surg 2021;47(2):214–26.

31. Fanous N. Correction of thin lips: "lip lift. Plast Reconstr Surg 1984;74(1):33–41.

32. Talei B. The modified upper lip lift: advanced approach with deep-plane release and secure suspension: 823-patient series. Facial Plast Surg Clin North Am 2019;27(3):385–98.

33. Weston GW, et al. Lifting lips: 28 years of experience using the direct excision approach to rejuvenating the aging mouth. Aesthet Surg J 2009;29(2):83–6.

34. Perkins SW, Balikian R. Treatment of perioral rhytids. Facial Plast Surg Clin North Am 2007;15(4):409–14, v.

35. Maloney BP. Cosmetic surgery of the lips. Facial Plast Surg 1996;12(3):265–78.

36. Chajchir A, Benzaquen I. Fat-grafting injection for soft-tissue augmentation. Plast Reconstr Surg 1989;84(6):921–34 [discussion: 935].

37. Gin I, et al. Treatment of upper lip wrinkles: a comparison of the 950 microsec dwell time carbon dioxide laser to manual tumescent dermabrasion. Dermatol Surg 1999;25(6):468–73 [discussion: 473-4].

38. Weissman O, et al. A new simple, safe, and easy solution for upper lip dermabrasion. J Drugs Dermatol 2012;11(5):649–52.

Minimally Invasive Techniques for Facial Rejuvenation Utilizing Polydioxanone Threads

Amit Kochhar, MD[a],*, Parvesh Kumar, BA[a], Kian Karimi, MD[b]

KEYWORDS

- Polydioxanone • Neocollagenesis • Thread-lifting • Complications • Barbed • Vector • Candidates

KEY POINTS

- Thread lifts offer a less invasive alternative to surgical lifts with fewer postoperative complications.
- Threads can be used to stimulate collagen production in the dermis/subdermis to give patients' skin a more rejuvenated appearance.
- Thread lifts are not suitable for all patients, and thus providers must ensure that they selectively offer these treatments to only ideal candidates with realistic expectations.

INTRODUCTION

Facial rejuvenation treatments countering the effects of aging have continued to gain popularity over the past few decades. More providers across multiple specialties are now offering treatments to improve skin elasticity, promote collagen production, contour facial structures, and increase skin volume. Although rhytidectomy is considered by surgeons to offer the greatest benefit for lifting tissues, it may also have significant complications, longer recovery times, and scarring in the subdermis and around the ears and submentum.[1] Thus, for patients who are more risk averse or do not want to go through the recovery or expense of surgery, thread-lifting treatments offer a minimally invasive procedure that may yield similar results with fewer complications and shorter recovery time.[2]

Thread lifting as a nonsurgical cosmetic procedure was first introduced by Sulamanidze and colleagues in 1990 to contour sagging facial tissue.[3] Since then, threading has advanced to treat fine wrinkles, skin laxity, nasolabial folds, crow's feet, smoker's lines, jawline structure, marionette lines,

tear trough regions, and submental fullness.[4] Polydioxanone (PDO) threads have two main mechanisms of action: either to lift desired facial anatomy for structural changes or to promote collagen and myofibroblast stimulation improving overall skin texture and health. These procedures are also commonly used in conjunction with complementary treatments such as dermal fillers, neuromodulators, and autologous blood platelet therapy such as platelet-rich plasma or platelet-rich fibrin. Thread-lifting has become a highly sought-out procedure and an effective, but temporary, alternative to surgical options.[5,6]

TYPES OF THREADS

Threads can be classified based on their direction, shape, absorbability, and chemical makeup. Threads can be unidirectional, bidirectional, or multidirectional, which describes the orientation of barbed projections on the threads. "Barbed" threads are suspension threads that engage the surrounding ptotic tissue and reposition superficial fat for accurate lifting. Bidirectional barbed threads do not require knots and have more

[a] Pacific Neuroscience Institute, 11645 Wilshire Boulevard, Suite 600, Los Angeles, CA 90025, USA; [b] Rejuva Medical Aesthetics, 1645 Wilshire Boulevard, Suite 605, Los Angeles, CA 90025, USA
* Corresponding author.
E-mail address: dramitkochhar@gmail.com

Facial Plast Surg Clin N Am 30 (2022) 375–387
https://doi.org/10.1016/j.fsc.2022.03.011
1064-7406/22/© 2022 Elsevier Inc. All rights reserved.

facialplastic.theclinics.com

A

B

C

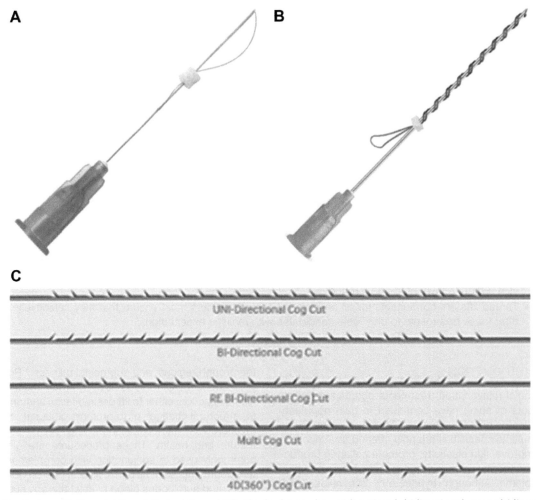

UNI-Directional Cog Cut

BI-Directional Cog Cut

RE BI-Directional Cog Cut

Multi Cog Cut

4D(360°) Cog Cut

Fig. 1. Smooth thread (A) and Barbed thread (B). The barbs can be unidirectional, bidirectional, or multidirectional (C). Bidirectional barbed threads will change directions in the middle of the thread.[3] (*From* Cobo R. Use of Polydioxanone Threads as an Alternative in Nonsurgical Procedures in Facial Rejuvenation. Facial Plast Surg. 2020 Aug;36(4):447-452. doi: https://doi.org/10.1055/s-0040-1714266. Epub 2020 Aug 31. PMID: 32866981. © Georg Thieme Verlag KG.)

consistent wound opposition compared with unidirectional threads. Sutures with knots have a higher risk of skin aggravation and scarring. Thus, bidirectional barbed threads may decrease the chances of these complications.[7] Most barbed threads have barbs on four to six sides of the threads, which increases the engagement of the threads to the tissue and provides a more reliable facial lift.[3] Barbed threads are usually inserted using a blunt cannula tip due to the lower risk of bruising, puncturing blood vessels, and injuring nerves.[8] "Molded barbed" threads are similar to barbed threads except they provide more stability and less slippage from the tissue. However, they are limited in that they are more difficult to remove whether there are any complications and thus are not used as regularly as their barbed counterparts.

Monofilament threads are "smooth threads" that do not have any barbs. They are best used for thin and crepey skin such as the neck, jawline, periocular region, and perioral region. These threads should be placed in the subdermis and not intradermally as they can cause an inflammatory response. "Twist" threads are oriented in a spiral around the needle applicator to promote neocollagenesis of thin and crepey skin. These threads, when placed near the vermillion border of the upper lip, stimulate collagen production and can provide a subtle lip enhancement (**Fig. 1**).[9]

Threads can also be categorized by being either nonabsorbable or absorbable. Nonabsorbable threads are not metabolized by the body and may need to be removed. Sulamanidze and colleagues originally used nonabsorbable barbed polypropylene antiptosis sutures (APTOSs) for nonsurgical facelifts.[10] However, these sutures had a high risk of complications such as scarring, nerve damage, and foreign body sensation.[11,12] Thus, thread-lifting treatments fell out of favor and resulted in a bad reputation across many specialties.[13]

However, in 2011, the development of absorbable threads gained popularity initially in Asia and Europe. These sutures have decreased risk of scarring and provide a more natural esthetic look, leading to higher patient satisfaction. The first absorbable threads used were polydioxanone (PDO) threads. PDO threads are monofilament threads that can be modified using laser technology to create unidirectional or bidirectional barbs.[5,14] These threads have high tensile strength, low tissue reactivity, high flexibility, and high durability.[9] Patients have reported sustained results between 6 and 18 months posttreatment. Poly-L-lactic acid (PLLA) threads are similar to PDO threads as they are absorbable threads, but they are more expensive and are more complicated to place. These threads, however, have sustained results between 12 and 18 months. The most recent absorbable threads approved by the Food and Drug Administration (FDA) are the polycaprolactone (PCL) threads. These threads are designed for smaller facial lifts and have results that can last up to 18 months.

ANATOMY

The skin is composed of three layers. The epidermis is the most superficial layer and is the main region for skin hydration. The next layer, the dermis, is the location of collagen and elastin, produced by fibroblasts. Collagen and elastin provide strength and elasticity for the skin, which leads to more skin tightness and less wrinkles. The deepest layer, the subcutaneous layer, provides insulation and is highly vascularized.

Threads are typically placed in the superficial subcutaneous planes. Monofilament threads are typically placed closer to the dermis, whereas barbed or suspension threads are placed more in the superficial subcutaneous plane. Anchoring suspension threads may be anchored on the deep temporal fascia (DTF).[9]

Absorbable threads are metabolized by the body through hydrolysis over a period of around 3–12 months that result in myofibroblast production, fibroblast production, increased vascularization, tissue contraction, and neocollagenesis. Neocollagenesis is the process of collagen formation in the dermal layer of the skin and myofibroblasts help with wound healing and contraction.[8,14,15]

THREAD PROCEDURES

Threads are mainly used as treatments for lifting the midface, lifting the lower third (jowls), brow lifting, neck rejuvenation, and collagen induction therapy. Barbed sutures are used during facial lifting procedures to engage the subdermal tissue and superficial fat pads while also repositioning them to the desired orientation. The barbs allow for better anchoring of the tissue compared with smooth threads. The barbed threads also induce fibrous tissue formation. Fibrous tissue helps keep the ptotic tissue in place after the skin has been lifted and thus sustains the facelift over longer periods. Histologic animal studies have demonstrated that the collagenesis and fibrous tissue formed by threads outlive the actual lifetime of the threads.[16] The sutures are placed along predetermined trajectories, or "vectors," and then are pulled in opposite directions to lift the sagging tissue. The most sought-out areas treated are the midface, the neck, the brow area, and the lower third of the neck.

Threads also stimulate neocollagenesis as they are broken down by the body under the skin. The goal for patients is to create a more rejuvenated and youthful appearance for patients. Histologic reviews of the skin after PDO threading have shown evidence for collagen thickening with type one and type three collagen formation.[3] Twist threads can be used as a hybrid treatment to provide both subtle lifting and stimulate neocollagenesis in areas such as the vermillion border.[8]

IDEAL CANDIDATES

Patient selection is crucial when determining ideal candidates for thread-lifting procedures as these procedures are not suitable for all people. It is important to stress to patients that thread lifting is only temporary and does not have as permanent or drastic effects as surgical intervention. Ideal candidates for facial thread lifts are between the ages of 30 and 50 with early signs of aging such as mild wrinkle formation, jowls, and decreased skin tightness. Ideal candidates also have thick skin, sufficient subcutaneous fat, strong bony projections, and flexible skin. Patients with too thin skin and insufficient subcutaneous fat increase the chances for postoperative complications and suboptimal results. Providers must also consider their medical history. Patients with underlying infections, compromised immune systems, keloid formation, diabetes, obesity, etc., should not be considered for threading treatments. Finally, providers must choose candidates with reasonable and attainable expectations (**Fig. 2**).[17]

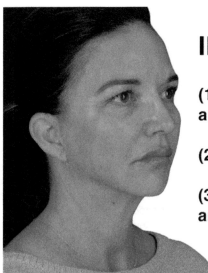

IDEAL CANDIDATE

(1) Sufficient Skin Thickness and Subcutaneous Fat

(2) Strong Bony Projections

(3) Skin of Sufficient Pliability and Mobility

Fig. 2. Characteristics of an ideal candidate for threading treatments. (*Courtesy of* Dr. Kian Karimi Rejuva Medical Aesthetics, Los Angeles.)

PREOPERATIVE PLANNING
Vector Planning

Vector planning is a useful tool to visualize planned treatments, make adjustments, and decrease mistakes. Although using a dermal marker, physicians will draw vectors from the insertion point to the end of the thread placement. Vector lines should be straight and can share the same insertion point but should not overlap.[18] For the midface, the zygomatic arch is typically used as the anchor and insertion point. The vectors will then extend along toward the oral commissure. For the lower third of the face and neck and temple regions, insertion points are near local ligaments to provide further stability (**Fig. 3**).

Materials

These materials are needed for threading treatment (**Fig. 4**).

- Topical anesthetic cream
- Lidocaine HCL 1% with epinephrine 1:1,000,000
- 1% Plain lidocaine
- 8.4% Sodium bicarbonate
- Suture scissors
- Forceps
- 18G needles
- 27G needles
- DermaSculpt 22 gauge 2 ¾" microcannula
- 3-mL syringes
- Tegaderm transparent film dressing 4′ x 4
- Disposable Chux
- Alcohol
- Peroxide
- Hibiclens antiseptic antimicrobial skin cleanser
- Ice packs
- 4x4 gauze
- Ultrasound gel

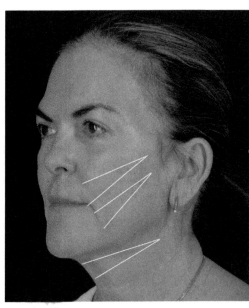

Fig. 3. Example of preoperative vector planning for thread lifting. (*Courtesy of* Dr. Kian Karimi Rejuva Medical Aesthetics, Los Angeles.)

Location	Pilot Needs (Barbs)	Size of Cannula (Barbs)	Barb Size	Pilot Needle (Molded)	Size of Cannula (Molded)
Lower 1/3	18G or 20G	18G or 21G x 90mm	4	18G	18G x 90mm
Midface	18G or 20G	18G or 21G x 90mm	4	18G	18G x 90mm
Brows	20G	21G x 60mm	4	18G	18G x 90mm
Neck	20G	21G x 90mm	4	18G	18G x 90mm

Fig. 4. Diagram showing the proper materials needed for different parts of the face for thread lifting.[8]. (*Data from* Karimi K, Chester CF, Reivitis A, Zhang E, Hunter A. Microcannula utilization for the injection of filler: standard of care? The American Journal of Cosmetic Surgery 2018: 35(4): 189-197.)

Pretreatment

Patients are advised to stop blood thinners 7 days before treatments as blood thinners can cause excessive bleeding during procedures. Patients should also stop smoking 2 weeks before procedures and stop drinking 3 days before treatments as both tobacco and alcohol can interfere in the healing process. Finally, patients should be well hydrated and have adequate sleep. Optionally, patients can take Arnica 2 days before treatments to help with any posttreatment edema and erythema.[19]

Photos and Consents

Photographs are important before and after treatments so patients can better visualize lifts of their facial structures and facial rejuvenation.[20] Pre-photo morphing using photo editing software is advised to give realistic expectations to the patient and to further plan out the procedure. Photos should be taken at multiple angles including the frontal view, bilateral profiles, and bilateral oblique positions. Two frontal photos should be taken with and without the patient smiling. Ensure that the patient is leveled with their head straight and any excess hair pushed behind their ears. It is important to make sure that there are not any unwanted

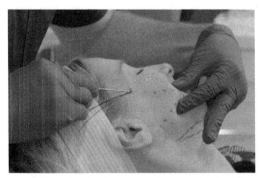

Fig. 5. Thread insertion on upper one-third of face. (*Courtesy of* Dr. Kian Karimi Rejuva Medical Aesthetics, Los Angeles.)

shadows on the patient's face to avoid unrealistic perceptions in the photos. Thus, adequate lighting and camera angles are essential to consider. Providers must also replicate these photos postoperatively for accurate comparisons.

Consent forms must be signed after thoroughly explaining expectations, risks, recovery, procedure techniques, and complications. Patients must understand that although thread lifting can provide similar results to surgical interventions, these procedures are temporary and routine follow-up procedures are needed for long-term effects. Consent forms should also indicate that there are no guarantees for the treatment, and the sutures may need to be removed.

OPERATIVE TECHNIQUES
Lifting

Once the patient has their planned vectors drawn on their face, consent forms signed, and photographs taken, the procedure can begin. The patient will be prepared by cleansing and sterilizing their face. The patient is then numbed with lidocaine HCL 1% with epinephrine 1:1,000,000 at each planned insertion point and allowed 10 minutes for the numbing to take effect. Although using a long 22 gauge $2^{3}/_{4}$ inch cannula inserted in the superficial subcutaneous plane along each vector, the face is further numbed with 2.5 mL of 1% plain lidocaine and 0.5 mL of sodium bicarbonate, 8.4%. The barbed threads are then fed into each cannula from the proximal to the distal end away from the insertion point (Fig. 5). Once the threads are placed along the vectors, the cannulas are slowly removed, thus engaging the tissue and lifting the sagging structures. It is during this part of the process that most of the irregularities such as skin dimpling can occur. However, the provider will also use their other hand to gently massage the face in the direction of the lift and aid in redraping the tissue in the correct position. Alternatively, if using an applicator instead of cannulas, the provider will also twist the end of the applicator handle to engage the tissue. After the

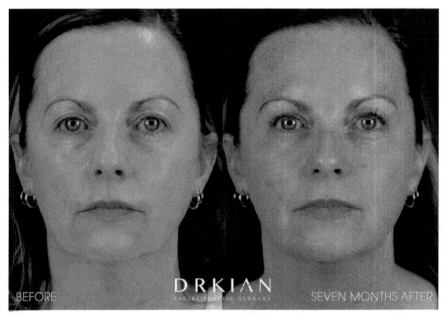

Fig. 6. Before and 7 months after thread lifting procedure. (*Courtesy of* Dr. Kian Karimi Rejuva Medical Aesthetics, Los Angeles.)

threads have been placed and the cannula or applicator removed, the physician will gently pull on the thread to make sure it is securely engaged. The thread will simply be pulled out if it is not. If the thread is pulled out, then the process is repeated with a new thread. Once the threads are securely engaged, the threads are cut making sure no threads are visible above the skin as the patient relaxes their face. More advanced techniques described recently will tie a knot between two threads, have the knot buried, and have the proximal segment of the thread rethreaded superolaterally and anchored on the DTF overlying the temporalis muscle. Finally, the face is massaged once more from the distal to the proximal end to ensure that the barbs are engaged and flat. This procedure takes between 30 and 60 minutes.[21] Fig. 6 shows a pre- and post-thread result.

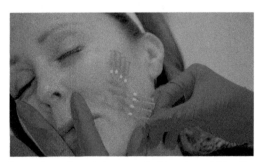

Fig. 7. Cannula matrix set up before thread insertion for collagen stimulation. (*Courtesy of* Dr. Kian Karimi Rejuva Medical Aesthetics, Los Angeles

MESH Procedure

Mesh procedures involve using smooth sutures to create a matrix in hollow parts of the face that will stimulate neocollagenesis and myofibroblast production. The mesh procedure is very similar to the lifting technique; however, the cannulas or applicators will remain in the skin throughout the procedure to determine where the threads have already been placed (Fig. 7). Once the matrix is created, the cannulas or applicators are then removed. In this technique, the face is not massaged in a certain direction since no lifting is occurring. The body then breaks down these threads stimulating collagen and myofibroblast production. Typically, six to nine threads are used for each jawline, five to ten threads for the jowl, and three to five threads for each temporal region.[3] Skin rejuvenation is usually first noted about 2 weeks after the procedure.[9]

POSTOPERATIVE CARE

Patients are advised to follow up 2 to 3 weeks after treatments. This allows enough time for postoperative edema and erythema to subside. In this interval, patients can apply cold compresses to the treated areas for 10 minutes every hour. The compresses will help reduce the expected swelling. Patients should also sleep elevated for the first 3 to 5 days and avoid exercise for a week. For pain, patients should take Arnica for 5 days postoperatively and take acetaminophen or ibuprofen

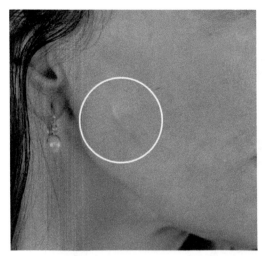

Fig. 8. Thread visualization through the skin. (*Courtesy of* Dr. Kian Karimi Rejuva Medical Aesthetics, Los Angeles

as needed.[19] Providers must stress to avoid any excessive facial expressions the week after treatment to prevent any displacement of the threads. Also, patients should avoid any facial massages or dental work for 1 month.[22] For general hygiene, patients are advised to wash their faces in the direction of the threads. Thus, it is important to review the procedure postoperatively and demonstrate proper cleaning techniques. Patients can return for their next thread appointment after a

minimum of 6 months. However, the threads have lasted up to a year for many patients. If patients are not satisfied and the provider deems "touch ups" are appropriate, then a thread treatment may be considered 3 months later. The provider may encounter fibrosis if placing additional threads where threads were placed previously. For patients considering rhytidectomy after placement of threads, it is recommended the patient delay surgical intervention for 6 to 12 months to allow for the reversal of the microfibrosis created by the threads.[9]

COMPLICATIONS

PDO threads may incur postprocedure complications that usually resolve with time but can still cause some concerns for patients. Thus, it is important to review all complications before treatments and before signing consent forms.

Common Postprocedural Complaints

Most patients after treatments should expect edema and swelling. The body's immune system naturally responded to wounds and punctures with inflammation. This usually subsides about 1 to 2 weeks after treatments.[23] Also, swelling occurs from the injected anesthesia fluid that the body will then break down. To help with the swelling, patients should ice the treatment areas three to four times per day. They can also take

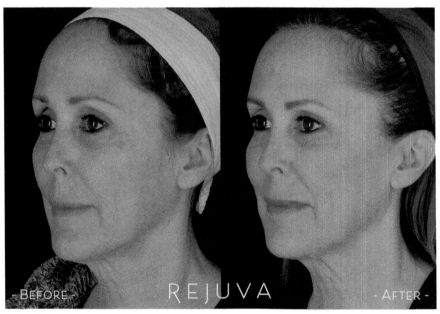

Fig. 9. Before and after left lateral view of a patient with threads and dermal fillers. (*Courtesy of* Dr. Kian Karimi Rejuva Medical Aesthetics, Los Angeles

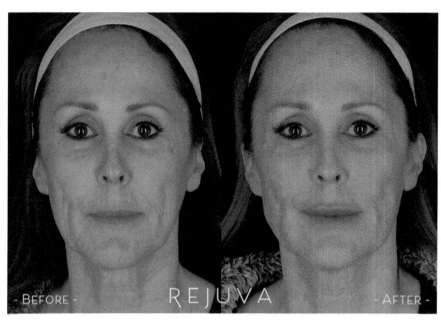

Fig. 10. Before and after frontal view of a patient with threads and dermal fillers. (*Courtesy of* Dr. Kian Karimi Rejuva Medical Aesthetics, Los Angeles

Arnica as a safe homeopathic method to reduce swelling post-treatment.[19]

Patients can also experience bleeding during and after treatments. To control the bleeding, blot and apply pressure using a sterile gauze to the area.[24] Excessive bleeding can occur but is rare. Thus, providers must have appropriate equipment and protocols ready if the bleeding is not easily controlled. Limiting blood thinner intake a week prior will not only limit the risk of excessive bleeding but will also limit the risk of unwanted errors during the procedure.[9]

Pain is common during and after treatments as well. Although patients are numbed with topical

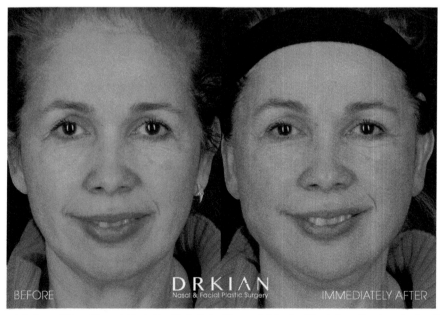

Fig. 11. Frontal view of NovaThreads Barb-5 with Infinity Plus and 1.0 mL of Restylane Contour to the Chin. (*Courtesy of* Dr. Kian Karimi Rejuva Medical Aesthetics, Los Angeles

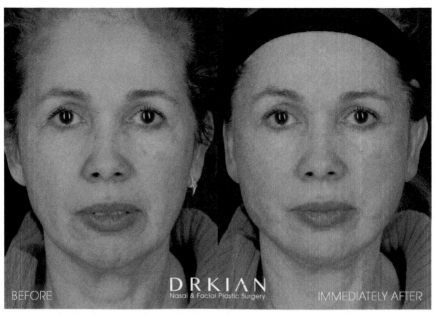

Fig. 12. Frontal view of NovaThreads Barb-5 with Infinity Plus and 1.0 mL of Restylane Contour to the Chin. (*Courtesy of* Dr. Kian Karimi Rejuva Medical Aesthetics, Los Angeles

and injected anesthetics, patients can still experience mild discomfort to sharp but short nerve pains. Patients can ice or take over-the-counter pain medications until symptoms resolve. In most cases, prescribed narcotics are not needed nor are recommended. In rare cases, the threads can be placed too deeply causing muscle pains for many weeks.

Patients may also experience bruising near the proximal insertion points. It is less common for patients to have bruising near the distal ends of the threads. Bruising will usually resolve by itself but can be aided with the use of icing and taking Arnica.

Finally, facial tenderness in the treatment areas is normal and common. However, patients should still avoid any excessive facial expressions 1 week

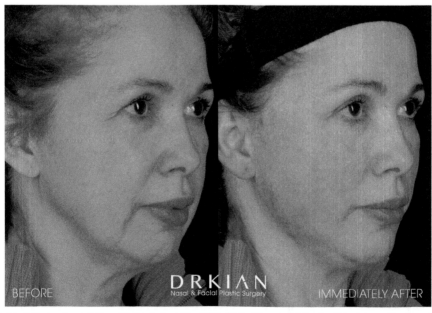

Fig. 13. Right oblique view of NovaThreads Barb-5 with Infinity Plus and 1.0 mL of Restylane Contour to the Chin. (*Courtesy of* Dr. Kian Karimi Rejuva Medical Aesthetics, Los Angeles

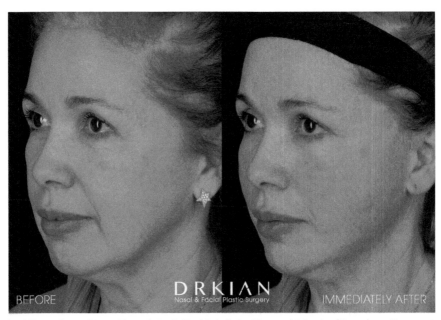

Fig. 14. Left oblique view of NovaThreads Barb-5 with Infinity Plus and 1.0 mL of Restylane Contour to the Chin. (*Courtesy of* Dr. Kian Karimi Rejuva Medical Aesthetics, Los Angeles

after treatments as they could compromise the positioning of the threads.

Complications

Threads can incite a foreign body response by the immune system if placed too superficially. Instead of breaking down the threads to stimulate neocollagenesis, the immune system within the dermis may instead try and push the threads out through the skin. This can cause an inflammatory event or visualization of the sutures through the skin. In the occurrence of this response, the threads must be removed and antibiotics may be prescribed to avoid possible infections.[25]

Threads may also be placed too superficially, which will cause a visual projection of the thread.

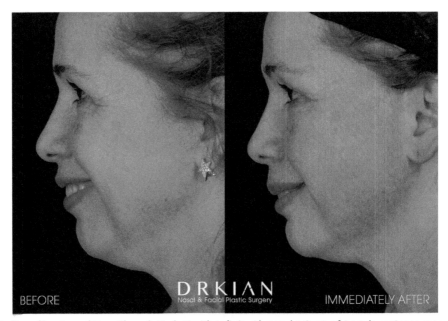

Fig. 15. Left profile view of NovaThreads Barb-5 with Infinity Plus and 1.0 mL of Restylane Contour to the Chin. (*Courtesy of* Dr. Kian Karimi Rejuva Medical Aesthetics, Los Angeles

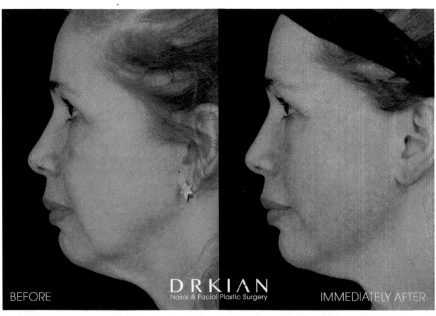

Fig. 16. Left profile view of NovaThreads Barb-5 with Infinity Plus and 1.0 mL of Restylane Contour to the Chin. (*Courtesy of* Dr. Kian Karimi Rejuva Medical Aesthetics, Los Angeles

These threads must be removed and replaced (Fig. 8).

The threads can create visual bumps on the patient's face that may be painful and aesthetically unpleasing to the patient. The patient can perform gentle upward massages to resolve these bumps, but in more severe cases the threads must be removed.[6,11]

There are cases where the threads cause facial asymmetry, typically due to one or more threads not having gripped the tissue fully. In these cases, additional threads may also be placed to attain the desired look. Most faces, however, are not naturally symmetric. Thus, minor asymmetry may be expected, and attempts at fixing it could cause further unwanted asymmetry.[14,25] Therefore, it is important to compare preoperative and postoperative photos to make an informed decision with patients to proceed with correcting any asymmetry.

Threads can also break and rip when under too much tension. If the desired lift is then lost due to this breakage, the physician may add another thread as a replacement. Otherwise, thread breakage does not pose as a major complication. The thread will still be broken down and stimulate neocollagenesis.[1]

COMPLEMENTARY PROCEDURES

Thread-lifting treatments can provide more natural rejuvenation than other modalities as they reposition ptotic tissues into a more youthful position. However, when paired with complementary treatments such as dermal fillers or neuromodulators, thread-lifting treatments are enhanced and patients are more satisfied.[26]

Thread lifting and dermal fillers are a perfect complement—threads lift ptotic tissues and fillers replace lost volume. Anecdotally, one of the authors (Dr. Kian Karimi) has found that when threads are used to lift the midface and lower third, the volume of dermal fillers typically required to achieve the desired outcome is cut in half. Thread-lifting treatments and dermal fillers are safe to use during the same appointment. However, the fillers should be used after threads have been placed to properly visualize the loss of volume and to prevent any interference with the engagement of the threads.[27] After dermal fillers and thread lifting treatments are finished, patients can also have neuromodulators injected to address any unwanted wrinkles.[28] These treatments are safe but must not be injected into the exact same place where the threads were placed to avoid interfering with the engagement of the threads (Figs. 9–16).

SUMMARY

The application of threads has evolved in the cosmetic realm of medicine and is a new tool in the esthetic armamentarium. Threads have become an important method to provide more natural-looking rejuvenation without the added potential complications of surgical intervention. However, threads are still limited in that only a select type of patient can actually have realistic benefits. Thread-lifts will continue to advance to provide a method for patients to achieve minimally invasive, safe, and effective ways to achieve natural facial rejuvenation.

CLINICS CARE POINTS

- Thread-lifting has become a highly sought-out procedure and an effective, but temporary, alternative to surgical options.

- Threads are used as treatments for lifting the midface, lifting the lower third (jowls), brow lifting, neck rejuvenation, and collagen induction therapy.

- Ideal candidates for facial thread lifts are between the ages of 30 and 50 with early signs of aging such as mild wrinkle formation, jowls, and decreased skin tightness.

DISCLOSURE

The authors have nothing to disclose.

REFERENCES

1. Tavares JP, Oliveira CA, Torres RP, et al. Facial thread lifting with suture suspension. Braz J Otorhinolaryngol 2017;83:712–9.
2. Shin JJ, Park TJ, Kim BY, et al. Comparative effects of various absorbable threads in a rat model. J Cosmet Laser Ther 2019;21(3):158–62.
3. Cobo R. Use of Polydioxanone Threads as an Alternative in Nonsurgical Procedures in Facial Rejuvenation. Facial Plast Surg 2020;36(4):447–52.
4. Kim CM, Kim BY, Hye Suh D, et al. The efficacy of powdered polydioxanone in terms of collagen production compared with poly-L-lactic acid in a murine model. J Cosmet Dermatol 2019;18(6):1893–8.
5. Tong LX, Rieder EA. Thread-Lifts: A double-edged suture? A comprehensive review of the literature. Dermatol Surg 2019;45:921–40.
6. Unal M, İslamoğlu GK, Ürün Unal G, et al. Experiences of barbed polydioxanone(PDO) cog thread for facial rejuvenation and our technique to prevent thread migration. J Dermatolog Treat 2019;1–4.
7. Einarsson JI, Vellinga TT, Twijnstra AR, et al. Bidirectional barbed suture: an evaluation of safety and clinical outcomes. JSLS : J Soc Laparoendoscopic Surgeons 2010;14(3):381–5.
8. Karimi K, Chester CF, Reivitis A, et al. Microcannula utilization for the injection of filler: standard of care? Am J Cosmet Surg 2018;35(4):189–97.
9. Karimi, K., & Khare, A. (n.d.). Resorbable Threads: Background, Types, Indications, and Techniques. Rejuva Medical Aesthetics.
10. Hochman M. Midface barbed suture lift. Facial Plast Surg Clin North Am 2007;15:201–207, vi.
11. Abraham RF, DeFatta RJ, Williams EF III. Thread-lift for facial rejuvenation: assessment of long-term results. Arch Facial Plast Surg 2009;11(3):178–83.
12. Rachel JD, Lack EB, Larson B. Incidence of complications and early recurrence in 29 patients after facial rejuvenation with barbed suture lifting. Dermatol Surg 2010;36(3):348–54.
13. Sulamanidze MA, Fournier PF, Paikidze TG, et al. Removal of facial soft tissue ptosis with special threads. Dermatol Surg 2002;28:367–71.
14. De Masi ECDJ, De Masi FDJ, De Masi RDJ. Suspension threads. Facial Plast Surg 2016;32:662–3.
15. Yoon JH, Kim SS, Oh SM, et al. Tissue changes over time after polydioxanone thread insertion: An animal study with pigs. J Cosmet Dermatol 2019;18(3):885–91.
16. Kim J, Zheng Z, Kim H, et al. Investigation on the Cutaneous Change Induced by Face-Lifting Monodirectional Barbed Polydioxanone Thread. Dermatol Surg 2017;43(1):74–80.
17. Shimizu Y, Terase K. Thread lift with absorbable monofilament threads. J Jpn Soc Aesthet Plast Surg 2013;35.
18. Lorenc ZP, Ablon G, Few J, et al. Expert Consensus on Achieving Optimal Outcomes With Absorbable Suspension Suture Technology for Tissue Repositioning and Facial Recontouring. J Drugs Dermatol 2018;17(6):647–55.
19. Stevinson C, Devaraj VS, Fountain-Barber A, et al. Homeopathic arnica for prevention of pain and bruising: randomized placebo-controlled trial in hand surgery. J R Soc Med 2003;96(2):60–5.
20. Lu SM, Bartlett SP. On facial asymmetry and self-perception. Plast Reconstr Surg 2014;133(6):873e–81e.
21. Karimi K. Technique for Nonsurgical Lifting Procedures Using Polydioxanone Threads. JAMA Facial Plast Surg 2018;20(6):511–2.
22. Kalra R. Use of barbed threads in facial rejuvenation. Indian J Plast Surg 2008;41(Suppl):S93–100.
23. Trayes KP, Studdiford JS, Pickle S, et al. Edema: diagnosis and management. Am Fam Physician 2013;88(2):102–10.
24. Glick JB, Kaur RR, Siegel D. Achieving hemostasis in dermatology-Part II: Topical hemostatic agents. Indian Dermatol Online J 2013;4(3):172–6.
25. Ahn SK, Choi HJ. Complication After PDO Threads Lift. J Craniofac Surg 2019;30(5):e467–9.
26. Ali YH. Two years' outcome of thread lifting with absorbable barbed PDO threads: Innovative score

for objective and subjective assessment. J Cosmet Laser Ther 2018;20(1):41–9.

27. Suárez-Vega D, Velazco de Maldonado G, García-Guevara V, et al. Microscopic and clinical evidence of the degradation of polydioxanone lifting threads in the presence of hyaluronic acid: a case report. Medwave 2019;19(1): e7575.

28. Satriyasa BK. Botulinum toxin (Botox) A for reducing the appearance of facial wrinkles: a literature review of clinical use and pharmacological aspect. Clin Cosmet Investig Dermatol 2019;12:223–8.

Microneedling-Associated Procedures to Enhance Facial Rejuvenation

Emily A. Spataro, MD[a],*, Kennedy Dierks[b,c], Paul J. Carniol, MD[d,1]

KEYWORDS

- Microneedling • Platelet-rich plasma • Radiofrequency • Skin resurfacing
- Collagen-induction therapy • Scar treatment • Facial rejuvenation

KEY POINTS

- Microneedling is a procedure in which small needles puncture the skin at various depths creating a mechanical injury that stimulates the wound-healing cascade and new collagen formation.
- Microneedling preserves the epidermis and is nonablative, which reduces inflammation, promotes more normal collage deposition rather than scar tissue, resulting in shorter downtime and fewer complications, especially in patients with darker skin.
- Indications for microneedling include acne scars, surgical or traumatic scars, melasma, striae/ stretch marks, androgenetic alopecia (with platelet-rich plasma [PRP] or minoxidil), alopecia areata (with steroids), skin rejuvenation, drug delivery of appropriate medications, radiofrequency delivery, and hyperhidrosis.
- Microneedling can also be used as a method to increase absorption of topical medications, growth factors, or PRP and deliver radiofrequency directly to the dermis.

INTRODUCTION

Microneedling, also referred to as percutaneous collagen induction therapy, is a method in which small needles puncture the skin to create a mechanical injury that stimulates the wound-healing cascade and new collagen formation. Other skin resurfacing techniques, such as laser resurfacing or chemical peels, injure both the dermal and epidermal layers of the skin, which can result in a longer healing process, as well as associated risks of dyschromia, scarring, and fibrosis. Microneedling preserves the epidermis and is minimally ablative to nonablative. This reduces inflammation and promotes more "normal" collage deposition.

Microneedling has a quicker recovery than most laser and superficial peels. In general, there is a low risk of complications, including in patients with higher Fitzpatrick skin types in whom there can be a greater risk of postprocedure pigmentation irregularities.[1–6] In addition to increasing collagen production in fibroblasts, microneedling also helps normalize the cell function of keratinocytes and melanocytes. It can be used as a method to increase absorption of topical medications and growth factors or deliver radiofrequency directly to the dermis.

HISTORY

Needling to induce scar tissue remodeling and collagen formation was first described by the method of subcision, which involves passing a needle under a scar or wrinkle to break up the scar and

[a] Division of Facial Plastic and Reconstructive Surgery, Department of Otolaryngology—Head and Neck Surgery, Washington University School of Medicine, St Louis, MO, USA; [b] Carniol Plastic Surgery, Summit, NJ, USA; [c] Joint Bachelor's/M.D. Program, Seton Hall University, 33 Overlook Road, Suite 401, Summit, South Orange, NJ 070901, USA; [d] Facial Plastic Surgery, Department of Otolaryngology Head and Neck Surgery, Rutgers New Jersey Medical School, Newark, NJ, USA
[1] Present address: 33 Overlook Road, Suite 401, Summit, NJ 070901.
* Corresponding author. 1044 North Mason Road, MOB #4, Suite L10, St Louis, MO 63141.
E-mail address: emily.spataro@wustl.edu

Facial Plast Surg Clin N Am 30 (2022) 389–397
https://doi.org/10.1016/j.fsc.2022.03.012

promote new collagen growth by inducing the wound healing cascade.[7] Later, tattoo devices without ink were used in a similar fashion, but the needles on these devices were too densely placed and resulted in overtreatment.[8] Rolling devices with needles less densely spaced compared with tattoo devices were introduced in 1996 by Fernandes, spurring more formal and consistent use of this method, which was termed percutaneous collagen induction.[9] The first dermal roller had needles of 3 mm in length, which limited its use in the office due to pain, and increased downtime due to ecchymosis and edema. However, studies using shorter needles of 1 mm were found to be just as effective in treating skin conditions while also significantly improving the amount of downtime and pain.[2,10] Electric-powered devices are now in wide use and compared with the manual rollers have the benefit of adjustable needle lengths that can be varied in the same treatment session, and improved pain tolerance from the vibration of the device on the skin.[11] Expanding on microneedling alone is the use of microneedling with adjuvant therapies such as platelet-rich plasma (PRP), other topical medications, and radiofrequency.

MECHANISM OF ACTION

Microneedling, in comparison to many other skin rejuvenation procedures, causes minimal damage to the epidermal layer of the skin, and only a small zone of injury in the papillary dermis to stimulate the wound healing cascade. Microneedling spurs a process of "scarless wound healing" with growth factors that are noninflammatory, namely transforming growth factor beta 3 (TNF-β3), rather than TNF-β1 and TNF-β2, which are more associated with inflammatory wound repair.[12,13] Additional growth factors released include platelet-derived growth factor (PDGF), connective tissue growth factor, epidermal growth factor (EGF), and fibroblast growth factor (FGF).[1] Histologic changes include increased epidermal thickness, increased collagen and elastin fibers, and increased presence of noninflammatory cytokines and growth factors, such as TNF-β3.[1,10,14] This process not only induces collagen formation from fibroblasts but also resets other dermal cell functions, such as normalizing the function of melanocytes, keratinocytes, and sebocytes and improves the strength of the dermal-epidermal junction.[15]

TYPES OF MICRONEEDLING
Cosmetic Microneedling

Cosmetic microneedling generally refers to rolling devices with needles between 0.2 and 0.3 mm in length, which do not penetrate the dermis. These rollers can be safely used by patients at home or estheticians and can augment medical microneedling performed in the office, other professional treatments, and skin care. Microneedling of the epidermis stimulates keratinocytes to release growth factors, which, in theory, stimulates cells in the dermis, including fibroblasts to create collagen, as well as improves the strength of the dermal-epidermal junction.[15] By creating channels in the epidermis, cosmetic microneedling also increases the absorption of topical skincare products by as much as 80%, thereby greatly increasing their efficacy.[16,17]

Medical Microneedling

Medical microneedling generally refers to needles of a length of 0.5 to 3 mm that breach the dermis. Injury at this depth induces the wound healing cascade previously discussed. Needle diameter is generally no more than 0.25 mm (corresponding to a 32 g needle), as sizes greater than this may cause scarring. The number of needles depends on the size of the roller or if an electric pen device is being used. A larger roller will have more needles, while electric pen devices come with a variety of options for the needle configuration. Many have an average of 12 needles in a circular pattern, but variable configurations are possible, with anywhere from 1 to 42 depending on the device (**Fig. 1**). Electric pens, unlike manual rollers, also have variable speeds, as well as an option of either battery power or corded power, which affects the maximum motor speed.[11] Some devices also have options of light-emitting diode (LED) light delivery, such as blue light to help treat acne.

Microneedling with Platelet Rich Plasma and Other Topical Agents

As stated previously, medical and cosmetic microneedling can also be used to increase the absorption of molecules too large to cross the skin's natural epidermal barrier. In particular, methods to increase growth factor delivery such as PRP, human stem cell-conditioned medium, other growth factor preparations, and medications such as minoxidil and tranexamic acid have been described.[18] It should be noted that all products infused with medical microneedling should be considered safe for systemic absorption, as allergic reaction and granuloma formation have been described after the use of topical products not meant for this purpose.[19]

PRP has been used with microneedling for both skin resurfacing purposes, as well as for hair growth. PRP is obtained by centrifuging patients'

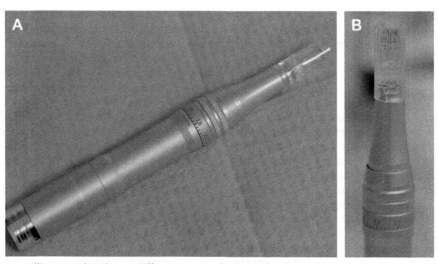

Fig. 1. Microneedling Pen. (*A, B*) Two different views of an electric microneedling pen. The disposable tip contains 12 needles, which can be set to different depths by turning the dial on the pen. Speed can also be adjusted.

blood to extract a platelet-rich layer, which contains growth factors such as PDGF, vascular endothelial growth factor (VEGF), EGF, TNF-β1, and TNF-β2, insulin-like growth factor-1 (IGF-1), and FGF. These growth factors then stimulate molecular signaling pathways to aid in skin and hair rejuvenation.[20–23] When injected, it is recommended to use an activator, such as calcium citrate; however, if PRP is microneedled into the skin, it is activated automatically and an activator is not required.[24] Although evidence is greatest in the benefit of PRP with microneedling to stimulate hair growth in androgenetic alopecia, it has also been shown to improve the appearance of atrophic acne scars compared with monotherapy alone or carbon dioxide laser.[25–32]

In addition to deriving growth factors from PRP, growth factor preparations from other sources, such as human stem cells, have been used, with the absorption of these large molecules into the skin facilitated by microneedling. Although sources such as adipocytes tend to be pro-inflammatory, ethical concerns surround embryonic or umbilical cord sources, and plant-derived stem cells are unlikely to have any effect on human cell regulation, preparations using lab-derived human recombinant growth factors are also being marketed for use in microneedling.[33] Although the specific growth factors in these preparations appear to be proprietary, they have been us with positive preliminary results with microneedling.[33]

Medications have also been used with microneedling to facilitate drug delivery. In particular, minoxidil has been used with hair loss to good effect.[34] Other uses include serums and tranexamic acid aimed at addressing pigmentation for

melasma.[35] It should be noted that as medical microneedling creates channels to the dermis that contains capillaries, any medication used in combination with medical microneedling should be approved for systemic absorption, as allergic reaction and granuloma formation has been reported with medications not designed for this purpose.[11,19] Cosmetic microneedling, which only penetrates the epidermis, has been used in combination with topical skincare products to increase absorption of these in the epidermis with good reported outcomes.[12]

Microneedling with Radiofrequency

Similar to facilitating drug or growth factor delivery directly to the dermis, microneedling can also be used as a method to deliver radiofrequency to the dermis while protecting the epidermis from thermal injury. By using microneedling devices with insulated needles and radiofrequency delivered at the tip of the needle, higher degrees of radiofrequency and thermal energy can be delivered to the dermis and subcutaneous tissue. The heat generated from the radiofrequency waves leads to collagen denaturation, causing contraction of the tissue, neocollagenesis, and tightening of the skin to improve skin laxity and wrinkles.[36–40] The most frequent use of radiofrequency microneedling (RFMN) is to treat acne scars in patients with darker skin types who are at high risk of post-inflammatory hyperpigmentation (PIH) with other modalities.[41–43] In studies comparing RFMN to bipolar radiofrequency, improved results were noted in acne scarring and aging skin.[44] Compared with fractionated laser resurfacing, similar improvements in acne scarring were found using RFMN but with decreased side effects.[45] It has also been applied to treat hyperhidrosis and rosacea.[46,47]

PREPROCEDURAL EVALUATION

Indications for microneedling include acne scars, surgical or traumatic scars, melasma, striae/stretch marks, androgenetic alopecia (with PRP or minoxidil), alopecia areata (with steroids), skin rejuvenation, drug delivery of appropriate medications, radiofrequency delivery, and hyperhidrosis.[11,48] Vascular lesions and some pigmented lesions are better addressed with other modalities such as intense pulsed light (IPL). Contraindications include active acne (although this is controversial and has been used in this setting with few complications), active local infections/viral infections, pustular rosacea, other open wounds from skin disorders such as psoriasis, severe solar keratosis, skin cancer, severe keloid risk, immunosuppression, recent neuromodulator or filler injection, or other recent skin resurfacing procedures.[11,48] It is recommended not to perform microneedling within 48 hours of neuromodulator treatments, as the increased perfusion may diminish its effect and distribute it beyond the injection site leading to potential complications. Likewise, it is recommended to avoid needling until 2 weeks after filler to reduce the risk of inflammatory reaction.

Patients should be assessed for anticoagulation use, and while not a contraindication, these medications increase the risk of bleeding or bruising after the procedure. Additionally, the use of medications that increase the photosensitivity of the skin should be assessed, especially in patients with darker skin, as this may increase the risk of PIH or other pigmentation issues postprocedure. More aggressive treatment (deeper or more passes) with the microneedle will also increase the risk of PIH in these patients although the risk is still significantly less than with lasers or peels. Although pregnancy is not a contraindication to microneedling, products that may be systemically absorbed, retinoids in particular, should not be used. Finally, a course of prophylactic antivirals should be considered in patients with a history of herpes simplex virus (HSV).[11]

TECHNICAL CONSIDERATIONS

When performing medical microneedling, the first step to achieving a comfortable experience for both patient and provider is appropriate anesthesia before the procedure. Many protocols to achieve this have been described, such as placement of topical lidocaine/prilocaine preparations, and benzocaine/lidocaine/tetracaine preparations. It should be noted that in preparations with a high concentration of lidocaine (such as 15% topical lidocaine), the maximal lidocaine dosage can be reached when this is applied over the whole face and neck and can result in cardiac toxicity.[11] Using compound formulas such as benzocaine 20%, lidocaine 6%, tetracaine 6% in a lipoderm base reduces this risk and provides effective anesthesia. Oral pain medication or nerve blocks can also be considered but are generally unnecessary if adequate time for absorption of the topical anesthetic is allowed (minimum of 10–15 minutes or as long as 30 minutes). It has also been suggested that cosmetic needling first will increase absorption of topical anesthetic, or the use of plastic wrap covering will enhance absorption. Finally, treatments with electric devices are generally less painful than roller devices of similar needle depths, as vibration diminishes the sensory nerve pain signals.[11,48]

Once the patient is appropriately anesthetized, the skin is then prepped with alcohol and microneedling commences. The depth of needle to be used depends both on the indication for microneedling, as well as the thickness of the skin in the treatment area. Electric pens with adjustable tips can generally be set to depths between 0.25 and 3 mm (see **Fig. 1**). Wrinkles, hyperpigmentation, and superficial scars can be adequately treated with needle depths between 0.5 and 1 mm, depths of 0.5 to 1.5 mm in the scalp for hair restoration, and deeper acne or hypertrophic scars, burns or stretch marks may require depths of 2 to 2.5 mm. Thin-skinned areas such as the periorbital areas likely do not require depths greater than 0.25 mm, the lip 0.5 mm, while thicker skin of the cheek likely requires depths of at least 1 mm. Using a depth of 3 mm will generally result in needle placement in the subcutaneous tissue, increasing the risk of complications.[11,48]

Once the appropriate depth of the needle is determined, the technique used involves holding the skin taught by stretching it with one hand and rolling or gliding over the skin. If using a manual dermal roller, this may require 15 to 20 passes in horizontal, vertical, and oblique directions applying equal pressure directed toward the outer border of the face and away from structure like the eyes and nose. Additionally, lighter pressures or speeds around areas of bony prominences like the zygoma or forehead should be used to decrease bruising risk. In areas of deep wrinkles, such as the nasolabial folds, the wrinkle should be stretched so the needles can make complete contact with the skin to avoid inadequately treating these areas. The manual roller can be used on dry skin or with a gliding medium such as hyaluronic acid. For electric devices, circular motions can also be used, and the use of hyaluronic acid as a gliding medium is recommended. If PRP is being used or other growth factor preparations, then this is used as the gliding medium. Repeated motion over the same area should be avoided to avoid track mark scarring. The desired endpoint should be diffuse, uniform erythema or pinpoint bleeding, and bleeding should be wiped away with saline-soaked gauze (Fig. 2).

Additional hyaluronic acid or PRP can be applied immediately after microneedling. Infusion of other topical products not meant for systemic absorption should be limited due to the risk of allergic reactions or granulomas. Other immediate postprocedure management includes LED treatments to reduce erythema and inflammation. Home care includes the resumption of most skincare products the following day, including makeup and sunscreen. For the first 3 to 5 days posttreatment, the skin will feel tight and dry, so more frequent use of moisturizers will counteract this. Home treatments that include the use of acids should be avoided for at least 2 weeks although enzyme peels can be used to minimize

inflammation and irritation of the skin about 5 days later. Cosmetic rollering can be resumed at this time point as well. As with most resurfacing procedures, patients should be counseled on minimizing sun exposure after treatment, and avoidance of photosensitizing medications.

Patients should be advised that the expected postprocedural course includes erythema for the first day, with the appearance of sunburnt skin (see Fig. 2). Bruising or petechiae can be present especially in patients with lighter, thinner skin in areas of bony prominences, or if aggressive treatment was used. Edema and exfoliation may occur over the next 2 to 3 days, but generally the skin returns to normal color after this amount of time.[11,48]

Optimal treatment regimens include a series of treatments repeated every 4 weeks for aging skin, every 14 days for hypertrophic scars, and every 2 months for depressed scars. Although every patient will require a different number of treatments, it is reasonable to counsel patients they may require anywhere from 3 to 6 treatments for optimal results, with one study reporting the best results after a series of four treatments.[10] It was also determined that the best results take a minimum of 12 to 24 weeks to become apparent and as long as 8 to 12 months after treatment.[49]

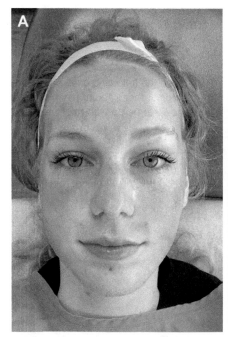
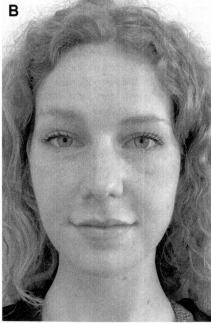

Fig. 2. Post-treatment expectations. (A) A patient who underwent microneedling immediately after the procedure with needle depths set at 0.3 mm for the chin, 0.5 mm for the forehead, and 1 mm for the cheeks. Note the skin erythema and pin-point bleeding. (B) shows this patient the following day with mild erythema present.

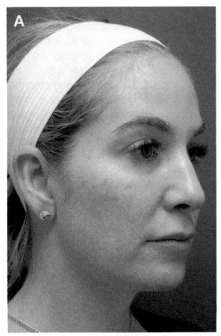
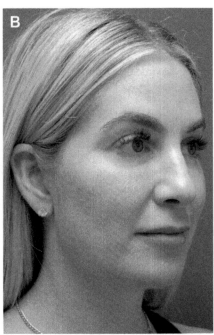

Fig. 3. Treatment of Acne scars. (*A*) A patient before a microneedling treatment for her acne scarring and pigmentation changes. (*B*) Her postprocedure results.

COMPLICATIONS

The most common complications of microneedling are pain during procedure, especially with greater depth of needle penetration, erythema, irritation, or mild edema.[19,48] Overly aggressive treatments, especially on areas of thinner skin, or over bony prominences, can cause bruising, petechiae, or track mark scarring.[50] Although rare compared with other skin resurfacing procedures, PIH has been reported in patients with an increased risk of photosensitization or sun exposure.[51,52] More recently, there have been increased reports of allergic reactions and granuloma formation due to the application of topical products during medical microneedling.[19] Patients with a history of herpes simplex should be cautioned about reactivation, and there is risk of superficial

infection as well, especially in immunocompromised patients.[11] We favor antiviral prophylaxis for patients with a history of facial herpes simplex. It is important that proper sterility and cleaning methods are used, particularly of nondisposable electronic devices, to reduce the risk of blood product exposure and cross-contamination.[11]

CASE STUDIES

Patients in the following case studies presented to the senior author's facial plastic surgery clinic to undergo treatments with microneedling or RFMN.

Acne Scars

The first patient presented with concerns about the appearance of acne scarring and pigmentation

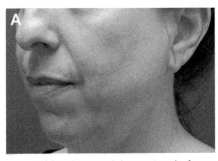
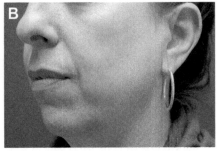

Fig. 4. Treatment of facial aging. (*A*) A patient before radiofrequency microneedling treatment for her facial aging. (*B*) Her postprocedure results.

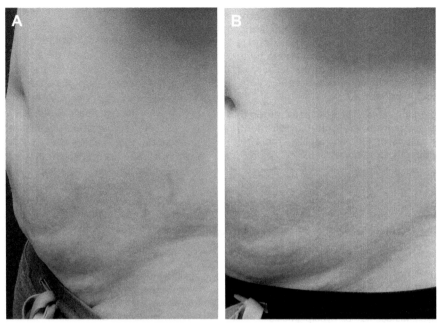

Fig. 5. Treatment of stretch marks. (*A*) A patient before her radiofrequency microneedling treatment for her stretch marks. (*B*) Her postprocedure results.

changes along her cheek, chin, and forehead as shown in **Fig. 3**A. She underwent microneedling treatment with an intensity of 50 for all areas and a depth of 0.4 mm along her chin, 0.7 mm along her forehead and 1.0 mm along her cheeks. Following a single procedure, she was satisfied with the cosmetic result of her acne scarring and skin pigmentation, with postprocedure results shown in **Fig. 3**B.

Facial Aging

The second patient presented with facial aging concerns, particularly of her nasolabial folds, jawline, and neck as shown in **Fig. 4**A. She underwent two treatments separated by 4 weeks of RFMN. The treatment protocol consisted of an intensity of 50, scan RF setting of 50, 1 pass, and depths of 1.3 mm for the jawline, 1.5 mm for the neck, and 1.6 mm for the chin. Her postprocedure results are shown in **Fig. 4**B.

Stretch Marks

The third patient presented with concerns of stretch marks on her abdomen as shown in **Fig. 5**A. She underwent four treatments separated by 4 weeks of RFMN. The treatment protocol consisted of an intensity of 70, depth of 2.5 mm, scan RF setting of 80, and 1 pass over the treatment area. Her postprocedure results are shown in **Fig. 5**B.

SUMMARY

Microneedling is a valuable tool clinicians can use in a variety of skin conditions to improve skin contour, laxity, and pigmentation. A primary benefit of this technique is its greater use in a variety of skin types, limited downtime, low cost, and minimal pain of the procedure. Associated treatments such as PRP, growth factor, medication, and radiofrequency delivery expanded the efficacy and applications of this modality as well. Although more research is needed to develop guidelines for the optimal use of microneedling, it has been shown to be an effective, safe, and versatile method for skin rejuvenation and resurfacing.

CLINICS CARE POINTS

- Microneedling uses small needles to puncture the skin at various depths creating a mechanical injury that stimulates the wound-healing cascade and new collagen formation.

- Microneedling preserves the epidermis and is non-ablative, which reduces inflammation, promotes more normal collage deposition rather than scar tissue, and results in shorter downtime and fewer complications, especially in patients with darker skin.

- Indications for microneedling include acne scars, surgical or traumatic scars, melasma, striae/stretch marks, androgenetic alopecia (with PRP or minoxidil), alopecia areata (with steroids), skin rejuvenation, drug delivery of appropriate medications, radiofrequency delivery, and hyperhidrosis.
- Microneedling can also be used as a method to increase absorption of topical medications, growth factors or PRP, and deliver radiofrequency directly to the dermis.

DISCLOSURE

The authors have nothing to disclose.

REFERENCES

1. Aust MC, Reimers K, Repenning C, et al. Percutaneous collagen induction: minimally invasive skin rejuvenation without risk of hyperpigmentation-fact or fiction? Plast Reconstr Surg 2008;122(5):1553e63.
2. Fernandes D, Signorini M. Combating photoaging with percutaneous collagen induction. Clin Dermatol 2008;26(2):192e9.
3. McCrudden MTC, McAlister E, Courtenay AJ, et al. Microneedle applications in improving skin appearance. Exp Dermatol 2015;24(8):561e6.
4. Elghblawi E. Intense retroauricular lymphadenopathy post-microneedling. J Cosmet Dermatol 2019; 18(6):2048–9.
5. Caccavale S, Iocco A, Pieretti G, et al. Curettage + microneedling + topical ALA-PDT for the treatment of acral resistant warts: our experience. Photodiagnosis Photodyn Ther 2019;27:276–9.
6. Dhurat R, Sharma A, Goren A, et al. Mission impossible: dermal delivery of growth factors via microneedling. Dermatol Ther 2019;32(3):e12897.
7. Orentreich DS, Orentreich N. Subcutaneous incisionless (subcision) surgery for the correction of depressed scars and wrinkles. Dermatol Surg 1995;21:543e9.
8. Doucet J. Needle dermabrasion. Aesthet Plast Surg 1993;1997:48e51.
9. Fernandes D. Percutaneous collagen induction: an alternative to laser resurfacing. Aesthet Surg J 2002;22:307e9.
10. Zeitter S, Sikora Z, Jahn S, et al. Microneedling: matching the results of medical needling and repetitive treatments to maximize potential for skin regeneration. Burns 2014;40(5):966e73.
11. Setterfield L. The concise guide to dermal needling – third medical edition – revised & expanded. 3rd edition. Acacia Dermacare; 2017.
12. Aust MC, Reimers K, Kaplan HM, et al. Percutaneous collagen induction-regeneration in place of cicatrisation? J Plast Reconstr Aesthet Surg 2011; 64(1):97e107.
13. Aust MC, Fernandes D, Kolokythas P, et al. Percutaneous collagen induction therapy: an alternative treatment for scars, wrinkles, and skin laxity. Plast Reconstr Surg 2008;121(4):1421–9.
14. Aust MC, Reimers K, Gohritz A, et al. Percutaneous collagen induction. Scarless skin rejuvenation: fact or fiction?: experimental dermatology concise report. Clin Exp Dermatol 2010;35:437e9.
15. Schmitt L, Marquardt Y, Amann P, et al. Comprehensive molecular characterization of microneedling therapy in a human three-dimensional skin model. PLoS One 2018;13(9):e0204318.
16. Stahl J, Wohlert M, Kietzmann M. Microneedle pretreatment enhances the percutaneous permeation of hydrophilic compounds with high melting points. BMC Pharmacol Toxicol 2012;13:5.
17. Serrano G, Almudéver P, Serrano JM, et al. Microneedling dilates the follicular infundibulum and increases transfollicular absorption of liposomal sepia melanin. Clin Cosmet Investig Dermatol 2015;8:313–8.
18. Ramaut L, Hoeksema H, Pirayesh A, et al. Microneedling: where do we stand now? A systematic review of the literature. J Plast Reconstr Aesthet Surg 2018; 71:1–14.
19. Soltani-Arabshahi R, Wong JW, Duffy KL, et al. Facial allergic granulomatous reaction and systemic hypersensitivity associated with microneedle therapy for skin rejuvenation. JAMA Dermatol 2014; 150:68e72.
20. Dhurat R, Sukesh M. Principles and methods of preparation of platelet-rich plasma: A review and author's perspective. J Cutan Aesthet Surg 2014;7:189–97.
21. Sánchez-González DJ, Méndez-Bolaina E, Trejo-Bahena NI. Platelet-rich plasma peptides: key for regeneration. Int J Pept 2012;2012:532519.
22. Steed DL. The role of growth factors in wound healing. Surg Clin North Am 1997;77:575–86.
23. Li ZJ, Choi HI, Choi DK, et al. Autologous platelet-rich plasma: a potential therapeutic tool for promoting hair growth. Dermatol Surg 2012;38:1040–6.
24. Cavallo C, Roffi A, Grigolo B, et al. Platelet-rich plasma: the choice of activation method affects the release of bioactive molecules. Biomed Res Int 2016;2016:6591717.
25. Jha AK, Vinay K, Zeeshan M, et al. Platelet-rich plasma and microneedling improves hair growth in patients of androgenetic alopecia when used as an adjuvant to minoxidil. J Cosmet Dermatol 2019; 18:1330–5.
26. Jha AK, Udayan UK, Roy PK, et al. Original article: Platelet-rich plasma with microneedling in androgenetic alopecia along with dermoscopic pre- and post-treatment evaluation. J Cosmet Dermatol 2018;17:313–8.

27. Shah KB, Shah AN, Solanki RB, et al. A comparative study of microneedling with platelet-rich plasma plus topical minoxidil (5%) and topical minoxidil (5%) alone in androgenetic alopecia. Int J Trichology 2017;9:14–8.

28. Greco J, Brandt R. The effects of autologous platelet rich plasma and various growth factors on non-transplanted miniaturized hair. Hair Transpl Forum Int 2009;19:49–50.

29. Escobar-Chávez JJ, Bonilla-Martínez D, Villegas-González MA, et al. A valuable physical enhancer to increase transdermal drug delivery. J Clin Pharmacol 2011;51:964–77.

30. Yepuri V, Venkataram M. Platelet-rich plasma with microneedling in androgenetic alopecia: study of efficacy of the treatment and number of sessions required. J Cutan Aesthet Surg 2021;14(2):184–90.

31. Hsieh TS, Chiu WK, Yang TF, et al. A meta-analysis of the evidence for assistant therapy with platelet-rich plasma for atrophic acne scars. Aesthet Plast Surg 2019;43:1615–23.

32. Long T, Gupta A, Ma S, et al. Platelet-rich plasma in noninvasive procedures for atrophic acne scars: a systematic review and meta-analysis. J Cosm Derm 2020;19(4):836–44.

33. Merati M, Woods C, Reznik N, et al. An assessment of microneedling with topical growth factors for facial skin rejuvenation: a randomized controlled trial. J Clin Aesthet Dermatol 2020;13(11):22–7.

34. Dhurat R, Sukesh M, Avhad G, et al. A randomized evaluator blinded study of effect of microneedling in androgenetic alopecia: a pilot study. Int J Trichology 2013;5(1):6–11.

35. Fabbrocini G, De Vita V, Fardella N, et al. Skin needling to enhance depigmenting serum penetration in the treatment of melasma. Plast Surg Int 2011;2011:158241.

36. Arnoczky SP, Aksan A. Thermal modification of connective tissues: basic science considerations and clinical implications. J Am Acad Orthop Surg 2000;8(5):305–13.

37. Zelickson BD, Kist D, Bernstein E, et al. Histological and ultrastructural evaluation of the effects of a radiofrequency-based nonablative dermal remodeling device: a pilot study. Arch Dermatol 2004;140(2):204–9.

38. Fitzpatrick R, Geronemus R, Goldberg D, et al. Multicenter study of noninvasive radiofrequency for periorbital tissue tightening. Lasers Surg Med 2003;33(4):232–42.

39. Alster TS, Tanzi E. Improvement of neck and cheek laxity with a nonablative radiofrequency device: a lifting experience. Dermatol Surg 2004;30:503–7.

40. Fritz M, Counters JT, Zelickson BD. Radiofrequency treatment for middle and lower face laxity. Arch Facial Plast Surg 2004;6(6):370–3.

41. Pudukadan D. Treatment of acne scars on darker skin types using a noninsulated smooth motion, electronically controlled radiofrequency microneedles treatment system. Dermatol Surg 2017;43(Suppl 1):S64–9.

42. Kim ST, Lee KH, Sim HJ, et al. Treatment of acne vulgaris with fractional radiofrequency microneedling. J Dermatol 2014;41(7):586–91.

43. Lee HS, Lee DH, Won CH, et al. Fractional rejuvenation using a novel bipolar radiofrequency system in Asian skin. Dermatol Surg 2011;37(11):1611–9.

44. Min S, Park SY, Yoon JY, et al. Comparison of fractional microneedling radiofrequency and bipolar radiofrequency on acne and acne scar and investigation of mechanism: comparative randomized controlled clinical trial. Arch Dermatol Res 2015;307(10):897–904.

45. Chae WS, Seong JY, Jung HN, et al. Comparative study on efficacy and safety of 1550 nm Er:Glass fractional laser and fractional radiofrequency microneedle device for facial atrophic acne scar. J Cosmet Dermatol 2015;14(2):100–6.

46. Kim M, Shin JY, Lee J, et al. Efficacy of fractional microneedle radiofrequency device in the treatment of primary axillary hyperhidrosis: a pilot study. Dermatology 2013;227:243–9.

47. Park SY, Kwon HH, Yoon JY, Min S, Suh DH. Clinical and Histologic Effects of Fractional Microneedling Radiofrequency Treatment on Rosacea. Dermatol Surg 2016 Dec;42(12):1362–9. https://doi.org/10.1097/DSS.0000000000000888. PMID: 27608206.

48. Alster TS, Graham PM. Microneedling: a review and practical guide. Dermatol Surg 2018;44(3):397–404.

49. Fabbrocini G, De Vita V, Monfrecola A, et al. Percutaneous collagen induction: an effective and safe treatment for postacne scarring in different skin phototypes. J Dermatolog Treat 2012;1:1e6.

50. Pahwa M, Pahwa P, Zaheer A. Tram track effect" after treatment of acne scars using a microneedling device. Dermatol Surg 2012;38:1107e8.

51. Asif M, Kanodia S, Singh K. Combined autologous platelet rich plasma with microneedling verses microneedling with distilled water in the treatment of atrophic acne scars: a concurrent split-face study. J Cosmet Dermatol 2016;15(4):434–43.

52. Majid I. Microneedling therapy in atrophic facial scars: an objective assessment. J Cutan Aesthet Surg 2009;2(1):26e30.

Nonsurgical Jaw Contouring
A Multi-Faceted Approach

Keon M. Parsa, MD[a],*, Michael Somenek, MD[b]

KEYWORDS

- Jaw line • Nonsurgical • Rejuvenation • Dermal fillers • Botulinum toxin • Deoxycholic acid
- Thread lift

KEY POINTS

- The loss of jawline definition with aging occurs as a result of bony resorption, fat repositioning, and increasing tissue laxity.
- Dermal fillers are the most common treatment modality used to define, sculpt, and shape the jawline through soft tissue envelope augmentation.
- Neurotoxins used to target hypertrophied muscles, particularly the masseter, can help give the jawline a slimmer and more defined appearance.
- Deoxycholic acid injections work by promoting lipolysis and can be particularly helpful when addressing fat accumulation in the submental area.
- Polydioxanone threads can be used to lift ptotic soft tissue around the jawline.

INTRODUCTION

The aging face is a function of facial volume loss resulting from a combination of factors, including bony resorption, fat repositioning, and overall tissue laxity. In the lower third of the face, these changes translate to loss of definition of the jawline. A well-contoured jawline is an aesthetically pleasing feature for both men and women. Studies have demonstrated that by improving jawline contour, one can help increase perceptions of attractiveness, likeability, extroversion, and masculinity/femininity.[1,2]

Rejuvenation of the jawline is now increasingly becoming part of routine aesthetic practice. Surgical procedures that help address the jawline and are associated lower face concerns include the use of facial implants, liposuction, fat transfer, and a variety of face and neck lifts. On the other hand, nonsurgical procedures continue to grow in popularity and are more commonly sought out

before proceeding with surgical intervention. As such, a comprehensive and multifaceted approach for nonsurgical jawline enhancement is key for practitioners in order to help optimize patient outcomes.

ANATOMY

A thorough understanding of the bony anatomy and surrounding neurovascular structures is vital when evaluating the jawline. As an aesthetic unit, the jawline is defined posteriorly by the extension of a line drawn from the helical attachment point at the temple to the anterior attachment of the lobule, anteriorly by a perpendicular line from the lower lip vermilion border, superiorly from the intertragal notch to the mental crease, and inferiorly by the inferior edge of the mandible.[3] The aesthetic units can be furthered subdivided into separate anatomic zones: masseteric, buccal, and mental (**Table 1**).

[a] Department of Otolaryngology/Head and Neck Surgery, MedStar Georgetown University Hospital, 3800 Reservoir Road Northwest, Washington, DC 20007, USA; [b] Somenek + Pittman MD, 2440 M Street Northwest, Suite 507, Washington, DC, USA
* Corresponding author.
E-mail address: keonparsa92@gmal.com

Facial Plast Surg Clin N Am 30 (2022) 399–406
https://doi.org/10.1016/j.fsc.2022.03.013
1064-7406/22/

Table 1
Overview of aesthetic zones of the jawline

Zone	Location	Subcutaneous	Vasculature	Nerves
Masseteric	Posterior to mandibular groove	Fat, musculoaponeurotic system, parotid gland, masseter muscle	Maxillary artery	Buccal and cervical branches of facial nerve
Buccal	Anterior to mandibular groove	Buccinator muscle, buccal fat	Facial artery, facial vein	Marginal mandibular branch of facial nerve
Mental	Anterior to prejowl sulcus	Mentalis muscle, depressor anguli oris muscle, depressor labii inferioris muscle	Submental artery, inferior labial artery	Mental nerve

The masseteric zone can be found posterior to the mandibular groove, which is found just anterior to the attachment of the masseter muscle. Moving from posterior to anterior within the masseteric zone, the skin transitions from thinner and finer to becoming thicker. Below the skin exists subcutaneous fat as well as the superficial musculoaponeurotic system. Several important deep structures can be found here, including the parotid gland and masseter muscle. The mandibular ramus, angle of mandible, and posterior third of the body fall within the masseteric zone.

The buccal zone can be found anterior to the mandibular groove and masseter muscle. This region is commonly identified as an area of concern for older patients owing to the development of jowls. Within this zone includes several important subcutaneous structures, such as the facial artery, facial vein and marginal mandibular nerve, buccal fat, and the buccinator muscles. The remaining portions of the mandibular body up to the parasymphysis are included within the buccal zone.

The mental zone is defined as the area anterior to a line connecting the oral commissure to the depression created by the mandibular ligament. This area contains the mental nerve as it exits through the mental foramen, branches of the facial and labial arteries, and several muscles, including the depressor anguli oris, depressor labii inferioris, and mentalis. Of note, the skin over the mentum is usually thick and firmly attached to the mentalis muscle. The parasymphysis and symphysis of the mandible are included within this zone.

Vasculature

The facial artery is a branch of the external carotid artery and is the major vessel supplying blood to the face. Knowledge of its location and course are therefore very important to avoid vascular complications, especially when injecting dermal filler. The facial artery can be palpated as it crosses the lateral border of the mandible anterior to the insertion of the masseter. The artery provides several branches as it courses superiorly including the inferior labial, superior labial, lateral nasal, and angular arteries.

Nerves

Distal nerve branches of the facial and trigeminal nerves should also be considered when performing nonsurgical procedures to augment the jawline. The facial nerve provides motor innervation to the muscles of facial expression, and the trigeminal nerve provides sensory innervation of the face. Of importance, patients with a history of trigeminal neuralgia may consider cosmetic interventions to the jawline as a trigger of recurrence. In addition, the use of lidocaine in this area can lead to a temporary paresis of facial musculature if distal branches of the facial nerve are affected.

EVALUATION

The aging process is highly variable between different individuals. The first step in advising a patient on the available options is to assess not only the patient's anatomy and overall facial appearance but also their expectations. As with any nonsurgical facial procedure, a careful aesthetic evaluation of the patient is important before suggesting an intervention. The aesthetic goal in jawline rejuvenation is to straighten the jawline, to smooth the transition between the mentum and the jowls, and to elevate the jowls in a posterosuperior vector to help restore definition and length.

In general, special focus should be given to the thickness/laxity of skin and subcutaneous tissue, prominence of the mandibular angle, jawline definition, chin projection and length, prejowl sulcus, cervical-mental angle, and the presence or absence of marionette lines.[4] Furthermore, parotid gland and masseter muscle hypertrophy are additional considerations that can impact the appearance of the jawline and should not be overlooked. Inherent asymmetries of the face and history of prior facial procedures should also be discussed. Last, patients should be examined at rest and in animation while in an upright position, as the soft tissue surrounding the jawline is relatively mobile and may shift depending on patient positioning.

Several key differences exist between women and men, which must be taken into account when performing jawline analysis. A youthful woman's face is often described as having the inverted triangle appearance, which occurs as the bizygomatic distance is wider than the bigonial distance. Preservation of this ideal should be maintained to avoid masculinizing the female face. In addition, the gonial angle tends to be more obtuse. Although the mandibular angle is generally less than 125° in both sexes, women tend to have a more obtuse angle than men by approximately 2.7°.[5] This difference helps create a softer transition from the mandibular body to ramus and a narrower width. As for the chin, female chins tend to be trapezoidal as well as shorter and thus can appear more pointed. Furthermore, the chin and lower jaw are typically shorter in women by as much as 20%.[6]

The aesthetic endpoint in men differs in that the male jaw is more angular and more prominent than women. This occurs because the mandible in men is larger and thicker with greater mandibular body height, especially at the symphysis. In contrast to women, the ideal bizygomatic to bigonial distance is approximately 1:1, whereas the gonial angle is more acute, contributing to a squarer-appearing jawline. Men also have more mandibular flare caused by masseteric attachments, contributing to the appearance of a wider jaw. In addition, the male mental subunit is wider, squarer, and longer than that of women. Last, the position of the male chin on profile view is in line with the lower lip vermilion or slightly anterior to this. Retrograde positioning whereby the chin is posterior to the lower lip vermilion can create a more feminine appearance.

NONSURGICAL TREATMENT OPTIONS

For patients who want to address the effects of an aging jawline as an alternative to a surgical procedure, there are several nonsurgical treatment options available. The approach to jawline rejuvenation and enhancement can include dermal fillers, chemodenervation with neuromodulators, deoxycholic acid injections, and polydioxanone

(PDO) threads. This section serves to address the different treatment modalities and aid in the decision-making process for optimal nonsurgical jawline rejuvenation.

Dermal Fillers

Dermal fillers have the ability to define, sculpt, and shape the jawline through soft tissue envelope augmentation. Not only do fillers work to help restore volume but also can help increase skin turgor to enhance results. The physicochemical structure of soft tissue fillers and their unique rheological properties play a pivotal role in determining how the filler behaves during and after injection. Two important properties that can be quantified are the viscosity and elasticity (G prime). The viscosity of a filler relates to how it flows from the needle, and the elasticity relates to the stiffness or ability to resist deformation during injection. The ability of a filler to lift soft tissue is directly related to the G prime. Thus, as the G prime increases, so does the firmness of the dermal filler. For jawline enhancement, using a filler with a higher G prime is preferred to provide more structure and support along the jaw. Noninvasive fillers that are most commonly used for jawline rejuvenation include calcium hydroxylapatite (CaHA), hyaluronic acid (HA), and poly-L-lactic acid (PLLA). Overall, the choice of filler for jawline is dependent on the subject's anatomy, injector, patient preference, and desired aesthetic outcome.

Calcium hydroxylapatite
CaHA is considered the workhorse for jawline contouring. CaHA is a biodegradable injectable that follows the same metabolic pathway as bone debris that occurs following bone fractures. The material is typically suspended in a methylcellulose carrier gel, which is composed of water, glycerin, and sodium carboxymethylcellulose. It is designed as a subdermal implant intended for volume enhancement. The typical expected duration for CaHA fillers is about 12 to 24 months. Although the filler does provide immediate volume to the jawline, the carboxymethylcellulose carrier is gradually resorbed over 2 to 3 months.

The ideal patient for CaHA injections includes those that require rigid structural augmentation. This can include individuals with thicker skin and soft tissue, a poorly defined mandible, and those with skin laxity requiring support to the overlying tissues. The patient in **Fig. 1** demonstrates the impact of CaHA injections for jawline rejuvenation.

Hyaluronic acid
HA is a glycosaminoglycan that is found naturally in the extracellular matrix of skin and is known to

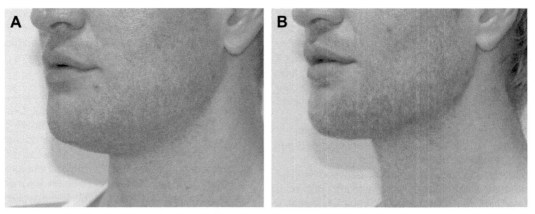

Fig. 1. Jawline contouring using 4 syringes of high G prime HA.A. Pre-treatment B. Post-treatment

be decreased on histopathologic evaluation of aged skin.[7] In comparison to CaHA fillers, HA fillers can have a duration of effect lasting 6 to 24 months, depending on the product choice and quantity injected. The highly hydrophilic nature of HA allows these fillers to volumize the face through this property, helping to improve skin turgor.

Although CaHA has a higher G prime than any HA filler, HA fillers can still be successfully used to augment the jawline. It is important to select an HA filler with a higher G prime to help achieve the desired outcome. The use of HA fillers is preferred for thin-skinned patients that desire a strong structural support, as this can provide a softer look to the overlying soft tissue envelope. The patient in **Fig. 2** demonstrates the impact of HA injections for jawline rejuvenation.

Poly-L-lactic acid

The last big class of facial filler that can be used for jawline rejuvenation is PLLA. This formulation contains particles of PLLA suspended in a carboxymethylcellulose and mannitol suspension. PLLA works to stimulate fibroblasts, which in turn produce collagen, similar to CaHA.[8,9] Unlike, CaHA and HA fillers, PLLA is used as a dermal stimulating agent more than a volumizing agent. The impact of PLLA is delayed compared with the others, with results that are progressive following the initial treatment and frequently more effective in a series of treatments. One advantage of PLLA fillers is longevity, with results lasting around 2 years. However, the authors believe that the effects of PLLA complement, rather than replace those of HA and CaHA filler.

Technique

Both needles and cannulas can be used for jawline and chin contouring, depending on the practitioners' level of comfort and overall preference. Using a cannula and a linear or angular approach can result in less overall trauma to the soft tissue, decreased bruising, and enhanced accuracy in filler placement. The decision to use needle versus cannula also has implications toward the depth of

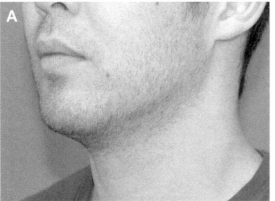
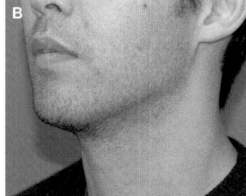

Fig. 2. Jawline and chin contouring with 3 syringes of CaHA. A. Pre-treatment B. Post-treatment

injection. When using needles, the target for injection is at the level of the mandibular periosteum. In contrast, the use of cannula can provide variability in depth of injection and in tissue planes, which can be advantageous when a multilayered injection is planned. Depending on the location, serial puncture, tunneling, and antegrade/retrograde linear threading are the most commonly used techniques, which can be used to safely and effectively enhance the contour and shape of these areas.

When using a cannula for jawline rejuvenation, a blunt-tip cannula is often used and is available in a variety of gauges, depending on the injector's preference. Injections are typically initiated posteriorly at the inferior edge of the angle of the mandible and continued medially using small aliquots of 0.05 to 0.1 mL per treatment area. As injections move medially, it is recommended to stay inferior to the masseter muscle. Care must be taken not to inject filler into the apex of the jowls, as this could potentially worsen the appearance of that region of the mandible. Injection volumes will vary with the location of the treatment site, the size of the area being treated, and individual patient characteristics. Overall, low-pressure, slow injections of small volumes with continuous movement is recommend to reduce the risk of complications. **Table 2** reviews the target depths of injection along the mandible.

Augmentation of the chin often requires injections in multiple layers. The order of injections starts with injection of the supraperiosteal plane to enhance the projection, length, and rotation of the mentum. Additional superficially placed injections can help fine tune overall appearance of the chin to reach the desired outcome. Special care must be taken to avoid the mental neurovascular bundle, which can be found approximately 1.5 cm superior to the mandibular border in this region.

Complications

The use of dermal fillers for jawline contouring is generally a safe and well-tolerated procedure.[8] Mild and transient symptoms, such as swelling, bruising, and erythema, after injection are not uncommon. Serious complications, on the other hand, are rare but important to highlight. Injectors must be aware of the risks of parotitis from intraglandular injection of dermal fillers. In addition, nodule or granuloma formation can occur with intramuscular injections. The most feared complication with dermal fillers is injection-related vascular compromise. Signs of vascular compromise include pallor, blanching, and severe pain the in the treated area, which can then progress to mottled discoloration or reactive hyperemia following injection. Progressive blue/black discoloration can occur over the next 24 to 48 hours, which can ultimately progress to necrosis,

Table 2
Target depth of injection based on area of jawline

	Depth of Injection
Preauricular area	Subcutaneous layer (lateral temporal fat compartment)
Angle of mandible	For male patients: supraperiosteal level to widen the face For female patients: subcutaneous layer to better define the angle
Body of mandible	Subcutaneous injections create a defined jawline appearance, whereas supraperiosteal injections are better used for older patients. A mixture of superficial and deep can also be used
Prejowl sulcus	Supraperiosteal level
Mentum	Supraperiosteal level. Additional superficial injections can be considered

ulceration, and skin breakdown if not properly addressed.[10] A thorough understanding of facial anatomy is key for injectors in order to prevent these complications.

Masseter Hypertrophy and Neuromodulators

The masseter muscle is a powerful superficial quadrangular muscle originating from the zygomatic arch and inserting along the angle and lateral surface of the mandibular ramus. It is one of the muscles of mastication, and its main function is to elevate the mandible during the closing of the mouth/jaw and clenching. Some patients, especially those who grind their teeth during sleep, can have a hypertrophied masseter. Asian patients are also more predisposed to having larger and hypertrophic masseter muscles.[11] The superficial fibers of the masseter can cause protrusion, resulting in a square jaw, wider face, and an overall masculinized appearance.

Masseter muscle hypertrophy and the resulting bulk can be reduced using neuromodulators. By relaxing the muscle and thereby reducing the thickness of it, a slimmer-appearing face (more V-shaped) can be achieved. This technique can also provide relief from the symptoms of clenching and teeth grinding. The typical dose of neurotoxin ranges between 10 and 25 units of botulinum toxin per side. A neuromodulator usually takes 2 weeks to take full effect when injected into other facial muscles, such as the frontalis and glabellar complex. However, in the case of masseter hypertrophy, the clinical effect of the neuromodulator can take 4 to 6 weeks to allow time for the muscle to atrophy. Similarly, the typical duration of neuromodulators is estimated to be 3 to 4 months, but a longer duration is commonly seen for masseter hypertrophy. This is thought to be due to the time it takes for the masseter to rehypertrophy.

Although uncommon, complications may occur with the use of neuromodulators to address masseter hypertrophy. One of the most common unwanted effects is a temporary decrease in mastication force given the impact on the masseter muscle and possible migration of neurotoxin to the surrounding muscles of mastication.[12] Given the proximity of the parotid, incidental injection of the gland may lead to xerostomia. Last, additional rare complications (<1%) that may occur include limitation in smile excursion owing to injection in the region of the risorius, subzygomatic volume loss, and paradoxic bulging.

Deoxycholic Acid

The presence of submental fat accumulation, referred to as a "double chin," is often associated with weight gain but can also be inherited. With aging, the deep fat compartments of the face (perioral, buccal fat) tend to atrophy and descend, whereas the superficial compartments (ie, submental, jowl regions) are more prone to hypertrophy. These volumetric changes contribute to fullness in the submental region and a subsequent loss of jawline definition.

For patients with excess submental fat, a fat-dissolving agent can be used. The active ingredient in fat-dissolving injections is deoxycholic acid, a secondary bile acid that helps with emulsification of fat. When injected in small volumes directly into the fat tissue, deoxycholic acid disrupts the fat tissue by dissolving the membranes of adipocytes (Fig. 3). The resulting glycerol and fatty acids are excreted through the lymphatic system. Although the body can regenerate fat cells, the process is very slow. Hence, the results from deoxycholic acid injections can be long lasting, especially if the patient continues to maintain a healthy lifestyle.

When used to address submental fat, deoxycholic acid is injected directly into the submental fat tissue. The typical dose is based on the total area being treated with the recommendation of 2 mg/cm^2.[13] Injections of 0.2 mL to 10 mL are spaced 1 cm apart using a prefabricated injection guide. Most patients undergo 2 to 4 treatment sessions to help optimize results.

The most frequent adverse events following deoxycholic acid injections to the submental area include edema, bruising, pain, and numbness at the treatment site. Several rarer complications have been reported, including skin necrosis secondary to intravascular injection, marginal mandibular nerve injury, dysphagia, and alopecia.[14]

Thread Lifting

Ptotic soft tissue can be repositioned with the help of facial threads. The goal of thread placement is to reposition the lower face fat compartments, in particular, the inferior jowl fat, middle and lateral cheek fat, and to restore jawline definition by suspending lax skin. For the jawline area, barbed threads in particular have proven to be effective.[15] When barbed sutures are used under the skin, they act to tighten and lift the loose areas of the face, creating better definition and contour. These threads are usually between 16 and 23 cm in length.[16] The length of thread used is often determined based on the severity of skin laxity, with longer threads providing a greater mechanical lifting effect.

PDO is a synthetic absorbable surgical suture that has been used in surgery for many years.

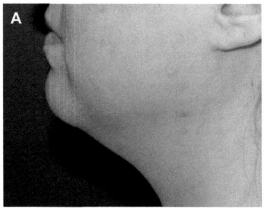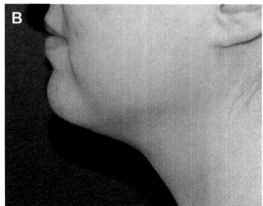

Fig. 3. Injection of 2 vials (4 mL–40 mg) of deoxycholic acid to submentum. A. Pre-treatment B. Post-treatment

The material is reabsorbed completely by the body in 4 to 6 months. This reabsorption is done by hydrolysis, triggering fibroblast production, which in turn produces more collagen in the targeted area.[17] In addition, following thread insertion, there is granulation tissue production and formation of fibrous tissue, which can help keep the ptotic tissue suspended. Studies have shown a statistically significant increase in volume immediately after treatment with variable efficacy up to 12 months.[18]

With the recent popularity of jawline thread lifting, there has been significant heterogeneity in techniques used. Although different techniques have been described, it is common to use more than one thread per side. The needle is inserted in the subcutaneous plane starting 1 cm above the mandibular angle and perpendicular to the skin surface. Once in the subcutaneous plane, the needle is then realigned at a 15° angle and advanced so that it is parallel to the skin with the goal of engaging the barbs in the fatty fibrous tissue. Following this, the distal end of the thread is pulled in the desired angle of suspension while gently pushing the skin in the opposite direction to fully engage the threads and provide a tissue lift. The ends of the thread are then cut at the skin.

One study found that the overall complication rate was roughly 34%.[18] The most common complications included migration and superficial displacement of the thread, infection, skin dimpling, and temporary facial stiffness. Additional research is required to elucidate the longevity and safety of this relatively new treatment modality.

SUMMARY

The jawline is key to the perception of attractiveness and youthfulness. Over time, a combination of mandibular bony resorption, facial fat repositioning and accumulation, as well as increased tissue laxity contributes to the loss of jawline definition. A thorough evaluation of each patient's preexisting anatomy and areas of deficiency is key to help determine the best treatment modality. In experienced hands, the use of dermal fillers, neuromodulators, deoxycholic acid, and thread lifting can be safe and effective with minimal side effects. A multifaceted approach has become an essential component of nonsurgical facial rejuvenation of the jawline.

DISCLOSURE

M. Somenek: No disclosures. K.M. Parsa: No disclosures.

CLINICS CARE POINTS

- The ability of a filler to lift soft tissue is directly related to the G prime. For jawline enhancement, using a filler with a higher G prime is preferred to provide more structure and support along the jaw.

- Deoxycholic acid disrupts fat tissue by dissolving the membranes of adipocytes, with the typical dose based on the total area being treated with the recommendation of 2 mg/cm². Injections of 0.2 mL to 10 mL are spaced 1 cm apart using a prefabricated injection guide.

- Facial threads can be used to reposition ptotic tissue with the length of thread used determined based on the severity of skin laxity. Longer threads provide a greater mechanical lifting effect.

REFERENCES

1. Reilly MJ, Tomsic JA, Fernandez SJ, et al. Effect of facial rejuvenation surgery on perceived

attractiveness, femininity, and personality. JAMA Facial Plast Surg 2015;17(3):202–7.

2. Parsa KM, Gao W, Lally J, et al. Evaluation of personality perception in men before and after facial cosmetic surgery. JAMA Facial Plast Surg 2019; 21(5):369–74.

3. Moradi A, Shirazi A, David R. Nonsurgical chin and jawline augmentation using calcium hydroxylapatite and hyaluronic acid fillers. Facial Plast Surg 2019; 35(2):140–8.

4. Buckingham ED, Glasgold R, Kontis T, et al. Volume rejuvenation of the lower third, perioral, and jawline. Facial Plast Surg 2015;31(1):70–9.

5. Hage JJ, Becking AG, de Graaf FH, et al. Gender-confirming facial surgery: considerations on the masculinity and femininity of faces. Plast Reconstr Surg 1997;99(7):1799–807.

6. Altman K. Facial feminization surgery: current state of the art. Int J Oral Maxillofac Surg 2012;41(8): 885–94.

7. Papakonstantinou E, Roth M, Karakiulakis G. Hyaluronic acid: a key molecule in skin aging. Dermatoendocrinol 2012;4(3):253–8.

8. Kim SA, Kim HS, Jung JW, et al. Poly-L-lactic acid increases collagen gene expression and synthesis in cultured dermal fibroblast (Hs68) through the p38 MAPK Pathway. Ann Dermatol 2019;31(1): 97–100.

9. Vazirnia A, Braz A, Fabi SG. Nonsurgical jawline rejuvenation using injectable fillers. J Cosmet Dermatol 2020;19(8):1940–7.

10. Sito G, Manzoni V, Sommariva R. Vascular complications after facial filler injection: a literature review and

meta-analysis. J Clin Aesthet Dermatol 2019;12(6): E65–72.

11. Cheng J, Hsu SH, McGee JS. Botulinum toxin injections for masseter reduction in East Asians. Dermatol Surg 2019;45(4):566–72.

12. Peng HP, Peng JH. Complications of botulinum toxin injection for masseter hypertrophy: incidence rate from 2036 treatments and summary of causes and preventions. J Cosmet Dermatol 2018;17(1):33–8.

13. Deeks ED. Deoxycholic acid: a review in submental fat contouring. Am J Clin Dermatol 2016;17(6): 701–7.

14. Farina GA, Cherubini K, de Figueiredo MAZ, et al. Deoxycholic acid in the submental fat reduction: a review of properties, adverse effects, and complications. J Cosmet Dermatol 2020;19(10):2497–504.

15. Preibisz L, Boulmé F, Paul Lorenc Z. Barbed polydioxanone sutures for face recontouring: six-month safety and effectiveness data supported by objective markerless tracking analysis. Aesthet Surg J 2022;42(1):NP41–54.

16. Wanitphakdeedecha R, Yan C, Ng JNC, et al. Absorbable barbed threads for lower facial soft-tissue repositioning in Asians. Dermatol Ther 2021; 11:1395–408.

17. Wong V, Rafiq N, Kalyan R, et al. Hanging by a thread: choosing the right thread for the right patient. J Dermat Cosmetol 2017;1(04):86–8.

18. Bertossi D, Botti G, Gualdi A, et al. Effectiveness, longevity, and complications of facelift by barbed suture insertion. Aesthet Surg J 2019;39(3):241–7.

Nonsurgical Rejuvenation of the Neck

Angela Sturm, MD[a,b,*], Tom Shokri, MD[c], Yadro Ducic, MD[d]

KEYWORDS

- Nonsurgical • Nonsurgical skin tightening • Neck tightening • Radiofrequency with microneedling

KEY POINTS

- The appropriate treatment should be one that addresses each patient's anatomy with the highest safety and efficacy.
- Radiofrequency with microneedling delivers energy precisely to stimulate collagen without risk of epidermal injury.
- Percutaneous radiofrequency delivers significantly higher power with greater energy than other energy devices directly to the fibroseptal network.

 Video content accompanies this article at http://www.facialplastic.theclinics.com.

INTRODUCTION

According to the 2018 American Society for Dermatology Surgery consumer survey on cosmetic and dermatologic procedures, 70% of respondents reported considering aesthetic procedures, which was up from 52% in 2014. Seventy-three percent was concerned with excess fat under the chin and neck, and the same percentage was concerned with skin texture, discoloration, or both.[1,2] Nonsurgical procedures have increased 508% from 1997 to 2015 with procedures for neck laxity one of the most popular.[3] Most patients wanted to look as young as they felt, to appear more attractive and to feel more confident. Patients are becoming more aware of treatments with easy accessibility of information on the Internet and social media. It is not only the baby-boomer generation seeking to minimize the signs of aging, but also the Generation X, Millennials, and even the Generation Z generations that are interested in nonsurgical interventions for rejuvenation and prevention. The younger generations are interested in procedures to postpone or obviate surgical facial rejuvenation.

AGING PROCESS

Aging of the neck has been called the "telltale" by some and is often forgotten in rejuvenation by the patient and at times by the medial professional. For these reasons, nonsurgical neck rejuvenation should be combined with facial rejuvenation for a uniform appearance in many cases. The neck has a complex network of the papillary and reticular dermis, fibroseptal network intermixed with subcutaneous fat and underlying fibrous fascia. The layers work in unison to create tone and quality.[4] Unlike the face that tends to lose volume, creating a more aged appearance, the neck may accumulate fat in the submental compartment, leading to loss of mandibular definition. Submandibular fat in the preplatysmal compartment may lead to an aged or overweight appearance.[5] Unlike fat accumulation in the body, neck laxity and fat redistribution cannot be improved with diet and

[a] Private Practice, 6750 West Loop South, Suite 1060, Bellaire, TX 77401, USA; [b] Department of Otolaryngology–Head and Neck Surgery, University of Texas Medical Branch, Galveston, TX, USA; [c] George Washington University, 2300 M Street, NW, 4th Floor, Washington, DC 20037, USA; [d] Private Practice, 4300 North Central Expressway #110, Dallas, TX 75206, USA
* Corresponding author. Private Practice, 6750 West Loop South, Suite 1060, Bellaire, TX 77401.
E-mail address: drsturm@drangelasturm.com

Facial Plast Surg Clin N Am 30 (2022) 407–417
https://doi.org/10.1016/j.fsc.2022.03.014
1064-7406/22/© 2022 Elsevier Inc. All rights reserved.

exercise and often is more severe after significant weight loss.[6] Just as in the face, the aging process involves not only gravitational descent but also photodamage leading to loss of collagen and elastin. Therefore, rejuvenation should address all of the applicable aspects of aging for that patient.

EVALUATION

Although a youthful neck can seem nebulous, specific criteria have been set. A youthful neck has a defined inferior mandibular border, visible sub-hyoid depression, visible thyroid cartilage bulge, visible anterior border of the sternocleidomastoid muscle, and a cervicomental angle of 105° to 120°.[7]

Evaluation of the patient should include the degree of preplatysmal and subplatysmal liposis, presence of platysmal bands, and degree of jowling extending into the neck. The location, course, and distance between the platysmal bands are noted. The patient should tense the platysma to evaluate if the bands are active or static.[8] Platysmal banding, possibly from weakening of the cervical fascia, can blunt the cervicomental angle and mandibular border, making it one of the factors that rapidly age a neck.[8]

Ideal patients for nonsurgical neck tightening include those who have skin neck laxity that is insufficient for a surgical facelift, those who do not ever desire a facelift, those who are not good surgical candidates from a medical perspective, and those that are trying to avoid surgery or delay surgery. Nonsurgical skin tightening is appealing for people who do not have the downtime for surgery because of a busy lifestyle. In addition, patients who are extremely risk averse may prefer nonsurgical treatment options because they have a lower risk profile. They are often willing to trade multiple treatments and less dramatic results for less downtime. Because nonsurgical options are, in general, less expensive than surgical options, these are preferred for the cost-conscious patient. Nonsurgical skin-tightening treatments can be performed in office with local anesthesia. Therefore, the patient does not have the cost or risks of general anesthesia or facility fees associated with a surgical procedure.

CONSIDERATIONS

As with any cosmetic procedure, the treatment should be tailored to that person's anatomy and goals, which could be a single treatment or a combination of treatments. Although liposuction is used in 81% of cases for submental fat reduction

and provides the most dramatic and reliable result, some patients do not desire surgical intervention because of resulting ecchymosis, skin laxity, recovery time, vascular or neurologic complications, cost, the potential for an unnatural result, or medical concerns.[9,10]

The mechanism of action of most skin tightening is based on the wound-healing cascade that occurs with surgical, thermal, or chemical trauma. The collagen contraction and skin tightening occur in the last phase of wound healing as the collagen is realigned.[11] This process takes at least 3 to 4 months to start to see results and can be up to 6 to 12 months. Multiple treatments are required for many of the modalities spaced between 4 and 8 weeks apart. Therefore, the process can take 6 months to complete the treatment series and then up to 6 to 12 months to see the final results. The results may be limited in patients with severe skin laxity, sun damage, or advanced age. The longevity of these treatments varies but can be from 1 to 5 years. With so many variables in the potential results, expectation management is key in the initial consultation.

THERAPEUTIC OPTIONS, OUTCOMES, AND COMPLICATIONS

The treatment plan for each patient may include a series of treatments, combination of treatments, or maintenance treatments. Key to deciding which modality to use is determining if the patient has lax skin, submental and submandibular fat, subplatysmal fat, or platysmal banding. Some of the options include neuromodulators, fractionated erbium:yttrium aluminum garnet (Er:YAG) or carbon dioxide (CO_2) laser, microneedling with radiofrequency, poly-L-lactic acid thread lifts, microfocused ultrasound, deoxycholic acid (DCA) injections, and percutaneous radiofrequency.

NEUROMODULATORS

Neuromodulators continue to be one of the most popular cosmetic procedures. From 2000 to 2018, the use of neurotoxins increased 800% with more than 7 million injections performed that year[12] and even grew 4.7% in 2021 during the COVID-19 pandemic.[13] Botulinum toxin is a neuromodulator produced by Clostridium botulinum, which blocks the release of acetylcholine from presynaptic vesicles at the neuromuscular junction, which relaxes the target muscle. Kane[14] is credited with introducing platysmal band neuromodulator injections in 1999. Brandt and Bellman[15] also published data about using neuromodulators for cosmetic treatments in the neck.

Although static platysmal banding can be improved, patients with dynamic platysmal banding and minimal skin laxity are ideal for neuromodulator injections. Because neuromodulators require routine maintenance and can achieve a smoother neck with increased definition in the jawline in the right patient, realistic expectations are critical for patient satisfaction.[8]

Once a thorough history and physical examination have been performed, botulinum toxin is injected directly into the anterior and lateral platysma. The bands should be grasped and distracted away from the neck to avoid injecting into and diffusion into deeper structures that could cause complications, such as dysphagia. Dosing can start from 10 to 30 units for women and 10 to 40 units for men using 2 to 12 injections points approximately every centimeter.[8] Other sources recommend injecting 5 to 10 units at each injection site at intervals of 1 to 1.5 cm using 50 to 100 total units on average, but up to 250 units if needed.[16]

In the study by Matarasso,[16] the best results were seen in the 80% of patients with mild to moderate platysmal bands and skin laxity, with 98.5% of the improvement judged as good to excellent by patients and physicians. Eighteen patients with the most severe platysmal bands did not respond to botulinum toxin. The onset of effect took up to 2 weeks and lasted 3 to 6 months. Bruising developed in 20% of patients, with 2 to 5 days of neck discomfort in less than 10%, neck weakness in 1%, and 2 weeks of dysphagia in 1 patient.[16,17] Other described complications include neck discomfort or the sensation of difficulty in pulling their head up from the pillow in the mornings.[18]

Levy[19] also described the "Nefertiti lift," in which approximately 10 units is injected along the mandibular border to improve jaw contour. The toxin counters the effect of the platysmal downward pull, usually in conjunction with injecting the depressor anguli oris. These injections are recommended to be no closer than 1 fingerbreadth below the mandibular border to prevent inadvertent effects on the muscles of mastication and lower lip depressors.[8]

MICROFOCUSED ULTRASOUND

Microfocused ultrasound was initially Food and Drug Administration (FDA) approved in 2009 with indications at the time of writing this article that include the brow, chin, neck, and chest. Ultrasound waves are focused at varying depths up to 4 mm with varying wavelengths to cause discrete focal heating of the dermis, subcutaneous fat, and superficial musculoaponeurotic system and to stimulate neocollagenesis and elastin

remodeling. The wavelengths pass through the epidermis, leaving the surface of the skin intact, leading to minimal to no downtime for the patient.[20]

The treatment can take up to 6 months to see a result and can be uncomfortable for some. In the study by Oni and colleagues,[20] 65.6% of patients saw improvement in their lower face and neck at 90 days. Blinded reviewers saw improvements in 58.1%. They reported pain scores of 6.09 in the submental area and 6.53 in the submandibular area. Local injections with lidocaine or oral anxiolytics have been required for patient comfort. Other side effects can include redness, bruising, and numbness that can last a couple of months.[20]

FRACTIONATED CARBON DIOXIDE TO THE NECK

Laser resurfacing has been a mainstay in facial rejuvenation for decades. Fractionated ablative lasers not only provide skin tightening during the alignment of collagen during the healing phase of the lasered areas but also improve pigmentation, texture, and sun damage, rejuvenating the neck in a more global sense. However, because of fewer pilosebaceous units in the neck compared with the face, complication rates are higher than facial procedures. Therefore, caution must be exercised in the treatment to avoid scarring and prolonged healing.[21–25]

Ablative laser resurfacing can be performed with ultrapulsed CO_2, ablative Er:YAG, and short pulse duration CO_2 laser. Tierney and Hanke[26] found fractionated ablative CO_2 to be effective and safe in rejuvenating the neck rhytids, skin texture, and laxity. In this study, on average 1.4 treatments at 6- to 8-week intervals were required for improvement of skin texture and laxity up to 59.3%. The Er:YAG laser is preferred for neck rejuvenation by some because of less thermal spread than CO_2, reducing healing time and potential complications, but potentially having less dramatic results. Goldman and colleagues[27] found a satisfaction rate of 51% with skin texture improvement of 39% by evaluations of nontreating physicians with Er:YAG.

Adverse events can include infection, scarring, koebnerization, dyschromia, contact dermatitis, prolonged erythema, acne, and milia. Contact dermatitis can be common and caused by a wide variety of creams and ointments. In particular, neomycin, bacitracin, and polymyxin can cause contact dermatitis and foreign body granulomas owing to its mineral oil content.[28,29] Even "natural" or "botanical" products can cause contact dermatitis despite patients perceiving them as gentle.[25] Although dyschromia is less common with fractionated CO_2 laser treatments, delayed-onset permanent hypopigmentation has been reported in up to 19% of cases.[21–23,30,31] Removing the intact skin barrier with the laser treatment allows for potential infection with bacteria, fungi, and viruses. The most dreaded adverse event is scarring, and most common cause of scarring is infection.[32,33] Manuskiatti and colleagues reported a 3.8% incidence of scarring.[34] In that series, every case was caused by infection, highlighting the importance of close monitoring of the healing process and prophylactic antibiotics, antifungals, and antivirals. Scarring can also occur from excessive fluence, density, passes, or pulse stacking.[35]

RADIOFREQUENCY WITH OR WITHOUT MICRONEEDLING

Radiofrequency has been used in medicine for more than 75 years and has been used for cautery, tightening of tissue for sleep apnea, and tumor destruction. Since 2002, dozens of radiofrequency devices have been approved to deliver energy to the dermis and fibroseptal network in the subcutaneous fat for cosmetic purposes. Because radiofrequency energy is independent of pigmentation, it can be used on all skin types. Patients with busy and active lifestyles appreciate the little to no downtime associated with these treatments.[36]

The delivery of radiofrequency can be monopolar or bipolar. In monopolar radiofrequency, the energy flows from an active electrode in the handpiece to a grounding pad placed elsewhere on the body. The advantage is that energy can be deposited deep in the dermis and fibroseptal network through a surface electrode. In bipolar radiofrequency, the energy flows between 2 adjacent electrodes both contained in the handpiece. The depth of penetration is postulated to be halfway between the electrodes.[37] Higher energies can be delivered with bipolar devices, but the energy cannot be delivered as deep.[36]

The initial radiofrequency devices pushed energy through the epidermis into the deeper layers with monopolar technology. The heat application was not precise, leading to inadvertent lipolysis and subdermal heating.[38] For safe radiofrequency treatments, the skin surface temperature must stay less than 42°C to 45°C because the threshold for epidermal burn is 44°C. To cool the skin, cryogen spray or constant motion was used. However, this can lead to inconsistent results owing to provider fatigue and uneven heating. Although there are mild benefits to heating the dermis to 45°C to 60°C, optimal results are achieved with temperatures of 65°C to 70°C, when coagulation, collagen denaturing, removal, and replacement

occur. Therefore, many transepidermal radiofrequency treatments have had variable and unimpressive results.[4]

Radiofrequency microneedling delivers the energy at the desired depths without risks associated with heating the epidermis. Insulated needles are used to pass through the epidermis down to 3 mm or more, which is deeper than what is safely achieved with lasers, where the dermis is heating to 65°C to 70°C. The insulated needles limit epidermal injuries to mechanical penetrations that are healed within 24 hours (Video 1). Some devices have noninsulated needles, which will result in larger radiofrequency thermal zones requiring longer healing times and increased risk of pigmentation changes. The wound-healing response critical for skin tightening, involving increased dermal thickness, cellularity, hyaluronic acid, and elastin content, has been shown to occur up to 10 weeks after the treatment.[39,40] Patient satisfaction can vary by device and by operator, but ranges from 72% to 90%[4] (Fig. 1). Radiofrequency with microneedling can safely be performed with topical applications of platelet-rich plasma or growth factors to speed healing, ablative or nonablative laser resurfacing to address surface pigmentation, or texture or soft tissue fillers to replace volume loss on the same day.[36,41] In general, the postprocedure downtime is minimal and averages 2 to 3 days. If higher energies are used, the downtime can be up to 1 week. Short-term complications include bruising, petechiae, acne flare, superficial infection, persistent "grid" marks, redness, edema, superficial burn, and postinflammatory hyperpigmentation. Long-term complications of scarring and textural abnormalities are extremely rare and usually due to provider technique.[36]

PERCUTANEOUS SKIN TIGHTENING WITH RADIOFREQUENCY

Subcutaneous and preplatysmal fat can create an obtuse cervicomental angle and contribute to an aged appearance. Submental liposuction has been the treatment of choice for submental liposis since the 1980s. Although it is a straightforward procedure, it can be associated with contour irregularities, postoperative edema, ecchymosis, and pain. Skin contraction after submental liposuction is only between 6% and 10% after 1 year, depending on the patient's skin elasticity. Therefore, submental liposuction can lead to the appearance of more laxity, irregularities, and inadequate skin contraction in some patients.[42–44] Percutaneous radiofrequency devices are able to ablate the subcutaneous fat and tighten overlying skin in ways

A 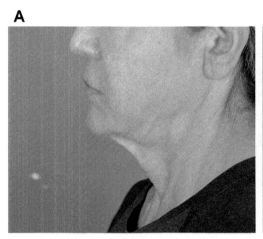 B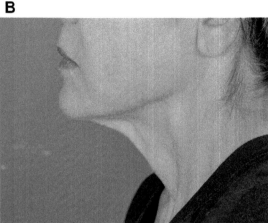

Fig. 1. Before (A) and after (B) photographs of a patient 3 months after undergoing microneedling with radiofrequency. The patient wanted to improve the laxity in her jowls and along her jawline. She also had improvement in her skin quality.

that have not been possible with other nonsurgical devices, providing a treatment option for patients with less than ideal skin turgor or over the age of 40 years who are not ideal candidates for submental liposuction alone, but are also not ideal facelift candidates.[45–49]

Percutaneous radiofrequency devices have a solid, blunt bipolar or monopolar probe that is passed in the subdermal space. The temperature is continuously monitored with an external electrode, treatment probe thermistor, or FLIR camera system and used to define treatment goals and durations. Tumescent anesthesia is critical in that the fluid aids in radiofrequency conductivity, creates space for the instrument to pass, and provides a secondary source of heat transfer after the application of the radiofrequency energy has been completed. The treatments have been shown to be safe and well tolerated under local anesthesia in the office (Video 2). After the completion of the treatment, a microliposuction cannula can be used to aspirate any liquefied fat from the treatment area to reduce potential posttreatment inflammation.[49]

Ideal patients have excess preplatysmal fat and mild skin laxity. Patients who are not ideal include those with subplatysmal fat without substantial preplatysmal fat, severe skin laxity, or marked platysmal banding. Unsuitable candidates include pregnant women, patients with collagen vascular disease, autoimmune diseases, acute infections, cochlear and neurostimulator implants, and patients who are medically unstable. Complications are not common but can include edema, erythema, tingling, seroma, hematoma, scarring, irregularities, and unacceptable aesthetic outcome. The direst complication of thermal injury

occurs in about 1% of cases. The procedure is well tolerated, and generally discomfort is controlled with over-the-counter analgesics.[49]

Percutaneous radiofrequency devices deliver significantly higher power with greater energy than other energy devices or laser-assisted liposuction. The deep adipose and fibroseptal network can be heated to higher temperatures without compromising the skin.[48] Studies show a 25% tissue contraction at 6 months and 35% to 60% tissue contraction at 1 year, significantly higher than liposuction alone or other skin-tightening technologies. [44,48,50–54] In an expert consensus panel and physician surveys, nearly 90% agreed that percutaneous radiofrequency can effectively and safely achieve skin tightening and fat reduction[55] (Fig. 2).

RADIOFREQUENCY-HELIUM PLASMA

Radiofrequency-helium plasma tightens submental and neck skin in the subdermal plane with minimal spread of the heat. Radiofrequency energy is delivered to the handpiece by the generator and is used to energize the electrode. When helium gas is passed over the energized electrode, a helium plasma is generated, which allows heat to be applied to tissue. The heat is generated by the actual production of the plasma by itself through the ionization and rapid neutralization of the helium atoms. Second, a portion of the radiofrequency energy used to energize the electrode and generate. Then, the plasma passes from the electrode to the patient and heats tissue by passing the current through the tissue. Subdermal tissues are heated to 65°C to 85°C for 0.040 to 0.080 seconds, which causes simultaneous tissue

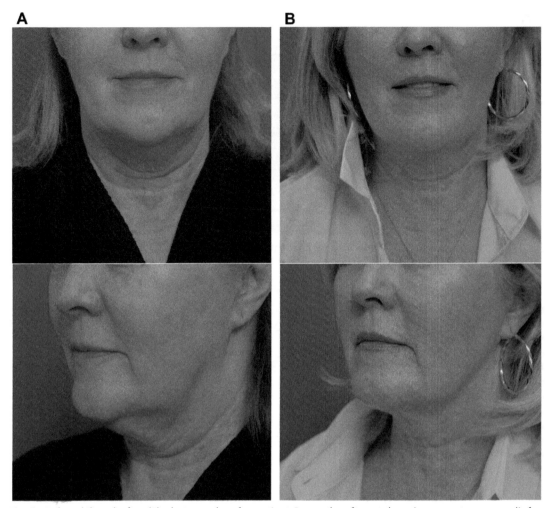

Fig. 2. Before (*A*) and after (*B*) photographs of a patient 3 months after undergoing percutaneous radiofrequency. The patient wanted to improve the laxity in her jowls, jawline, and neck. She was not interested in excisional surgery, so was very pleased with her results and not having general anesthesia.

desiccation and protein denaturation leading to coagulation targeting the fibroseptal network.[11] Ruff and colleagues[56] reviewed charts, finding a patient satisfaction rating of 74% and that 68% would consider having their procedure repeated. Risks include pain, bleeding, scarring, infection, and seroma, particularly if performed with excessive energy in the fascial planes.

DEOXYCHOLIC ACID

DCA was the first lipolytic substance approved by the FDA for fat reduction in the submental area in 2015. The investigation into DCA started in 2007 as a nonsurgical option to submental liposuction. DCA is a secondary bile acid that functions to emulsify and solubilize dietary fats to facilitate absorption into the gastrointestinal tract. The

pharmaceutical industry developed synthetic DCA with identical chemical structure, but no contaminants of human or animal origin.[57,58] When injected into the preplatysmal fat in the submental region, DCA causes rupture of adipocyte cell membranes, leakage of cytoplasmic content, lysis, and subsequent inflammatory response dominated by neutrophils.[59–61] On the seventh day after injection, macrophages scavenge the cell debris and lipids.[59,61–63] On day 28, fibroblasts are recruited, and there is remission of the inflammation. A series of up to 6 injections is recommended every 4 weeks.[61,62,64,65] Ascher and colleagues[58] found more than 1 point improvement in the Clinician-Reported Submental Fat Rating Scale in 62.3% of patients and patient satisfaction of 64.8% compared with 29.3% in placebo. Patient-reported secondary efficacy endpoints showed improvements in submental fat severity and perceived self-image.

Contraindications include infection at the site of injection, pregnancy, or age less than 18 years. One of the more concerning complications is paresthesia of the marginal mandibular nerve that is usually mild to moderate and transient from the temporary demyelination and inflammation of the nerve. Other adverse effects include edema (87%), bruising (72%), pain (70%), numbness (66%), and induration (23%). Local pruritis and nodules may also occur.[59,66–68] The events range from mild to moderate in severity and are generally transient. Adverse reactions that occur less frequently include dysphagia, damage to lymph nodes, salivary glands, and muscles, neutrophilic dermatosis, submental abscess, and nerve injury.[69] Beard alopecia has been reported as transient or permanent with pathologic condition consistent with nonscarring alopecia, which may be due to the inflammatory response. Skin necrosis has been described and could be from intra-arterial injection, vasoconstrictive effects, disruption of cell membranes and tissue inflammation, or intradermal injection.[70–73] The reported adverse events include some that have dire consequences and permanent effects. Therefore, the use of DCA requires a series of precautions, post-injection care, detailed knowledge of anatomy, skin preparation for the injections, and expectation management.

CRYOLIPOLYSIS

Cryolipolysis has been shown to reduce subcutaneous fat safely and effectively by cooling the skin and fat to a temperature that causes lipolysis but does not damage the skin. Fat is more susceptible to cold injury compared with water-rich epidermal and dermal cells.[74] Cryolipolysis has FDA clearance for safe and effective removal of fat in the submental area in addition to the flanks, abdomen, thighs, back, bra area, under the buttocks, and arms. The most aesthetically pleasing results have been found with multiple cryolipolysis applicators with overlap in the midline and repeated sessions spaced 6 weeks apart.[74]

Bernstein and Bloom[74] showed a statistically significant reduction in fat thickness and skin surface area as well as having high patient satisfaction (93%), higher than the previous study of 83%.[74,75] Objectively, quantified image analysis found a 2.7% reduction in mean surface area, which was used to quantify skin tightening.[75] Adverse events are generally mild and included erythema, edema, bruising, and self-resolving numbness and tingling. Injury to the marginal mandibular nerve is possible but was not seen in this study.[74]

FUTURE DIRECTIONS

Nonsurgical skin tightening is an ever-evolving field. The demand for more dramatic results with less downtime will continue to drive the field and available technology. For the foreseeable future, the physician and patient will have to continually evaluate the risk profile, potential outcome, downtime, and cost of each procedure in relation to the option of surgery, as no current noninvasive procedure can deliver surgical results. However, each generation of skin tightening technology becomes more efficacious and more directed and has less downtime. The trend will only continue. Combining treatments to address not only laxity but also sun damage and textural changes will continue to be the way of the future, as well. It is already commonplace to combine microfocused ultrasound with soft tissue filler or microneedling with radiofrequency and fractionated nonablative laser resurfacing for tightening, collagen stimulation, and texture improvements. The option to be a surgeon in the aesthetic field without knowledge of or interest in noninvasive technology is a thing of the past. Patients desire noninvasive options to surgery, as well to maintain their surgical investments.

DISCUSSION

In the annual Plastic Surgery Statistics report published by the American Society for Plastic Surgery, more than 13 million minimally invasive cosmetic procedures were performed in 2020, and this market has grown by 174% from 2000 to 2020. Face and neck procedures make up most of the minimally invasive procedures.[76]

Patients are presenting at younger ages for rejuvenation with 49% of cosmetic procedures performed on adults aged 20 to 54 years old.[76] This younger generation takes 25,000 selfies in their lifetime, making them more aware of their appearance, particularly their neck profile, than ever before.[53] Social media is not only a way that we see ourself at every angle but is also a source of information always at our fingertips about new procedures, making cosmetic procedures more accessible and desirable. Providing noninvasive treatment options allows surgeons to build relationships with younger patients, making the lifetime value of each patient greater. These are patients that will return for other nonsurgical procedures and then eventually facial rejuvenation surgery when they are ready. In 2018, 45% of people who underwent cosmetic procedures had already undergone a surgical or nonsurgical cosmetic procedure.[77]

Options exist for every patient's anatomy and goals. Patients with minimal laxity and dynamic platysmal bands benefit from neurotoxin. Patients with mild to moderate skin laxity may benefit from microneedling with radiofrequency or microfocused ultrasound. Extensive sun damage with skin laxity can be corrected with ablative fractional lasers. Percutaneous radiofrequency, percutaneous helium plasma, DCA, and cryolipolysis are all suitable for patients with subcutaneous, preplatysmal fat and mild skin laxity. Patient satisfaction, scientifically proven results, and low complication rates are important to evaluate when choosing a treatment for a patient or device to purchase. Noninvasive skin tightening can be combined with medical grade skin care, cosmetic injections, and skin treatments, such as peels or laser resurfacing, leading to higher patient satisfaction and recurring revenue for the practice. Skin-tightening treatments can also be viewed as part of a maintenance program for patients who have undergone facial cosmetic surgery.

SUMMARY

Nonsurgical neck tightening can deliver dramatic, noticeable results by stimulating collagen using heat energy and the healing process. With detailed assessment and diagnosis of each patient, treatment plans can be optimized to each patient. Low downtime options that avoid general anesthesia and directly address each person's anatomy and aspects that age the neck lead to satisfied, returning patients.

CLINICS CARE POINTS

- A youthful neck has a defined inferior mandibular border, visible subhyoid depression, visible thyroid cartilage bulge, visible anterior border of the sternocleidomastoid muscle, and a cervicomental angle of 105° to 120°.
- Evaluation of the patient should include the degree of preplatysmal and subplatysmal liposis, presence of platysmal bands, and degree of jowling extending into the neck.
- Patients with dynamic platysmal banding and minimal skin laxity are ideal for neuromodulator injections.

- Microfocused ultrasound has a patient satisfaction of 65.5% but can be painful for patients and takes time to see results.
- Fractional ablative lasers dramatically tighten the skin, resurface rhytids, and improve sun-damaged skin, but can have complications if not performed carefully.
- Radiofrequency microneedling safely delivers energy for tissue contracture at various depths with coated needles resulting in high patient satisfaction rates.
- Percutaneous radiofrequency devices deliver more energy and have more skin contraction than any other device or laser-assisted liposuction with low complication rates.
- Helium plasma and radiofrequency precisely deliver heat but have limited scientific studies.
- Deoxycholic acid is the first lipolytic injection but can be associated with more potential adverse events.
- Cryolipolysis freezes adipocytes at temperatures that do not damage skin.

DISCLOSURE

Dr A. Sturm is a Luminary for Lutronic USA for devices unrelated to this content. The authors have no conflicts of interest relevant to the content of this article.

SUPPLEMENTARY DATA

Supplementary data related to this article can be found online at https://doi.org/10.1016/j.fsc.2022.03.014.

REFERENCES

1. American Society for Dermatology Surgery Consumer Survey 2018.
2. American Society for Dermatology Surgery Consumer Survey 2014.
3. IAPAM. Aesthetic trends in 2019 & 2018 according to the IAPAM. Available at: https://iapam.com/aesthetic-trends-2019-iapam.html. Accessed October 29, 2021.
4. Locketz GD, Bloom JD. Percutaneous radiofrequency technologies for the lower face and neckfacial. Plast Surg Clin North Am 2019;27(3):305–20.
5. Hatef DA, Koshy JC, Sandoval SE, et al. The submental fat compartment of the neck. Semin Plast Surg 2009;23(4):288–91.
6. Park JH, Kim JI, Park HJ, et al. Evaluation of safety and efficacy of non-invasive radiofrequency

technology for submental rejuvenation. Lasers Med Sci 2016;31(8):1599–605.

7. Ellenbogen R, Karlin JV. Visual criteria for success in restoring the youthful neck. Plast Reconstr Surg 1980;66(6):826–37.

8. Rohrich RJ, Savetsky IL, Cohen JM, et al. Effective treatment of platysmal bands with neurotoxin. Plast Reconstr Surg Glob Open 2020;8(6):e2812.

9. Jianu DM, Filipescu M, Jianu SA, et al. The synergy between lasers and adipose surgery in face and neck rejuvenation: a new approach from personal experience. Laser Ther 2012;21(3):215–22.

10. Schlessinger J, Weiss SR, Jewell M, et al. Perceptions and practices in submental fat treatment: a survey of physicians and patients. Skinmed 2013;11(1):27–31.

11. Richard D.Gentile MD, MBAab Renuvion/J-plasma for subdermal skin tightening facial contouring and skin rejuvenation of the face and neck. Facial Plastic Surgery Clinics of North America Volume 27, Issue 3, August, Pages 273-290

12. Aesthetic Plastic Surgery National Databank Statistics 2020 Aesthet Surg J, Volume 41, Suppl_2, 2021, Pages 1–16.

13. American Society for Aesthetic Plastic Surgery (ASAPS) 2021 Cosmetic Surgery National Data Bank Statistics.

14. Kane MA. Nonsurgical treatment of platysma bands with injection of botulinum toxin A. Plast Reconstr Surg 1999;103:656–63.

15. Brandt FS, Bellman B. Cosmetic use of botulinum A exotoxin for the aging neck. Dermatol Surg 1998;24(11):1232–4.

16. Matarasso A, et al. Botulinum A exotoxin for the management of platysma bands. Plast Reconstr Surg 1999;103:645–52.

17. GJ Hruza, reviewing Matarasso A et al. Botox Platysmal Bandsplast Reconstr Surg 1999 Apr 1, 1999

18. Tamura BM. The effect of botulinum toxin on the platysma muscle. Curr Derm Rep 2012;1:89–95.

19. Levy PM. The "Nefertiti lift": a new technique for specific recontouring of the jawline. J Cosmet Laser Ther 2007;9(4):249–55.

20. Oni G, Hoxworth R, Teotia S, et al. Kenkel evaluation of a microfocused ultrasound system for improving skin laxity and tightening in the lower face. Aesthet Surg J 2014;34(7):1099–110.

21. Ward PD, Baker SR. Long-term results of carbon dioxide laser resurfacing of the face. Arch Facial Plast Surg 2008;104:238–43 [discussion: 244–245].

22. Bernstein LJ, Kauvar AN, Grossman MC, et al. The short- and long-term side effects of carbon dioxide laser resurfacing. Dermatol Surg 1997;23(7):519–25.

23. Bisson MA, Grover R, Grobbelaar AO. Long-term results of facial rejuvenation by carbon dioxide laser resurfacing using a quantitative method of assessment. Br J Plast Surg 2002;55(8):652–6.

24. Avram MM, Tope WD, Yu T, et al. Hypertrophic scarring of the neck following ablative fractional carbon dioxide laser resurfacing. Lasers Surg Med 2009;41(3):185–8.

25. William MR. Fractional CO2 laser resurfacing complications. Semin Plast Surg 2012;26(3):137–40.

26. Tierney EP, Hanke CW. Ablative fractionated CO2, laser resurfacing for the neck: prospective study and review of the literature. J Drugs Dermatol 2009;8(8):723–31.

27. Goldman MP, Fitzpatrick RE, Manuskiatti W. Laser resurfacing of the neck with the erbium:YAG laser. Dermatol Surg 1999;25(3):164–8.

28. Fisher A. A. Lasers and allergic contact dermatitis to topical antibiotics, with particular reference to bacitracin. Cutis 1996;58(4):252–254.8.

29. Lee S. New and unresolved complications after upper lid blepharoplasty and full face CO2 laser resurfacing. Paper presented at: the 20th Annual Scientific Meeting of the American Academy of Cosmetic Surgery; January 29–Feburary 2, 2004; Hollywood, FL.

30. Laws RA, Finley EM, McCollough ML, et al. Alabaster skin after carbon dioxide laser resurfacing with histologic correlation. Dermatol Surg 1998;24(6):633–6.

31. Shamsaldeen O, Peterson JD, Goldman MP. The adverse events of deep fractional CO(2): a retrospective study of 490 treatments in 374 patients. Lasers Surg Med 2011;43(6):453–6.

32. Ross RB, Spencer J. Scarring and persistent erythema after fractionated ablative CO2 laser resurfacing. J Drugs Dermatol 2008;7(11):1072–3.

33. Fife DJ, Fitzpatrick RE, Zachary CB. Complications of fractional CO2 laser resurfacing: four cases. Lasers Surg Med 2009;41(3):179–84.

34. Manuskiatti W, Fitzpatrick RE, Goldman MP. Long-term effectiveness and side effects of carbon dioxide laser resurfacing for photoaged facial skin. J Am Acad Dermatol 1999;40(3):401–11.

35. Choi B, Barton J, Chan E, et al. Infrared imaging of CO2 laser ablation: implications for laser skin resurfacing. Proc SPIE 1998;3245:344–51.

36. Weiner SF. Radiofrequency microneedling: overview of technology, advantages, differences in devices, studies, and indications facial. Plast Surg Clin North Am 2019;27(3):291–303.

37. Sadick NS, Makino Y. Selective electro-thermolysis in aesthetic medicine: a review. Lasers Surg Med 2004;34:91–7.

38. De Felipe I, Del Cueto SR, Perez E, et al. Adverse reactions after nonablative radiofrequency: follow-up of 290 patients. J Cosmet Dermatol 2007;6(3):163–6.

39. Hantash BM, Renton B, Berkowitz RL, et al. Pilot clinical study of a novel minimally invasive bipolar microneedle radiofrequency device. Lasers Surg Med 2009;41(2):87–95.

40. Hantash BM, Ubeid AA, Chang H, et al. Bipolar fractional radiofrequency treatment induces neoelastogenesis and neocollagenesis. Lasers Surg Med 2009;41(1):1–9.

41. Calderhead G. Combining microneedle fractional radiofrequency and LED photoactivation. Prime 2014;2(6):15–23.

42. Locketz GD, Bloom JD. Percutaneous radiofrequency lower face and neck tightening technique. JAMA Facial Plast Surg 2018. https://doi.org/10.1001/jamafacial.2018.0917.

43. Kim YH, Cha SM, Naidu S, et al. Analysis of postoperative complications for superficial liposuction: a review of 2398 cases. Plast Reconstr Surg 2011; 127(2):863–71.

44. Gasparotti M. Superficial liposuction: a new application of the technique for aged and flaccid skin. Aesthetic Plast Surg 1992;16(2):141–53.

45. Key DJ. Comprehensive thermoregulation for the purpose of skin tightening using a novel radiofrequency treatment device: a preliminary report. J Drugs Dermatol 2014;13(2):185–9.

46. Key DJ. Integration of thermal imaging with subsurface radiofrequency thermistor heating for the purpose of skin tightening and contour improvement: a retrospective review of clinical efficacy. J Drugs Dermatol 2014;13(12):1485–9.

47. Paul M, Mulholland RS. A new approach for adipose tissue treatment and body contouring using radiofrequency-assisted liposuction. Aesthet Plast Surg 2009;33(5):687–94. 4.

48. Paul M, Blugerman G, Kreindel M, et al. Three-dimensional radiofrequency tissue tightening: a proposed mechanism and applications for body contouring. Aesthet Plast Surg 2011;35(1):87–95.

49. Locketz GD, Bloom JD. Percutaneous radiofrequency technologies for the lower face and neck. Facial Plast Surg Clin North Am 2019;27(3):305–20.

50. Mulholland RS. Nonexcisional, minimally invasive rejuvenation of the neck. Clin Plast Surg 2014; 41(1):11–3.

51. Mulholland RS. Radio frequency energy for noninvasive and minimally invasive skin tightening. Clin Plast Surg 2011;38(8):437–48.

52. DiBernardo B. Journal JR-A surgery, 2009 undefined. Preliminary report: evaluation of skin tightening after laser-assisted liposuction. Available at: academic.oup.com. Accessed November 4, 2018.

53. Theodorou SJ, Del Vecchio D, Chia CT. Soft tissue contraction in body contouring with radiofrequency-assisted liposuction: a treatment gap solution. Aesthet Surg J 2018;38(Suppl_2): S74–83.

54. Duncan DI. Nonexcisional tissue tightening. Aesthet Surg J 2013;33(8):1154–66.

55. Kinney BM, Andriessen A, DiBernardo BE, et al. Use of a controlled subdermal radio frequency thermistor for treating the aging neck: consensus recommendations. J Cosmet Laser Ther 2017; 19(8):444–50.

56. Ruff PG, Doolabh V, Zimmerman EM, et al. Safety and efficacy of helium plasma for subdermal coagulation. Dermatol Rev 2020;1:108–14.

57. Fagien S, McChesney P, Subramanian M, et al. Prevention and management of injection related adverse effects in facial aesthetics: considerations for ATX-101. (deoxycholic acid injection) treatment. Dermatol Surg 2016;42:S300–4.

58. Ascher B, Fellman J, Monheit G. ATX-101 (deoxycholic acid injection) for reduction of submental fat. Expert Rev Clin Pharmacol 2016;9(9):1131–43.

59. Walker P, Lee. A phase 1 pharmacokinetic study of ATX-101: serum lipids and adipokines following synthetic deoxycholic acid injections. J Cosmet Dermatol 2015;14(1):33–9.

60. Rotunda AM, Weiss SR, Rivkin LS. Randomized double-blind clinical trial of subcutaneously injected deoxycholate versus a phosphatidylcholine-deoxycholate combination for the reduction of submental fat. Dermatol Surg 2009;35(5):792–803.

61. Dayan SH, Humphrey S, Jones DH, et al. Overview of ATX-101 (deoxycholic acid injection): a nonsurgical approach for reduction of submental fat. Dermatol Surg 2016;42:S263–70.

62. Georgensen C, Lipner SR. The development, evidence and current use of ATX-101 for the treatment of submental fat. J Cosmet Dermatol 2017;16(2): 174–9.

63. Thuantong R, Bentow JJ, Knopp K, et al. Tissue-selective effects of injected deoxycholate. Dermatol Surg 2010;36(6):899–908.

64. Rotunda AM, Suzuki H, Moy RL, et al. Detergent effects of sodium deoxycholate are a major feature of an injectable phosphatidylcholine formulation used for localized fat dissolution. Dermatol Surg 2004; 30(7):1001–8.

65. Goodman G, Lee D, Smith K, et al. Reduction of submental fat with ATX-101: a pooled analysis of two international multicenter double-blind, randomized, placebo controlled studies. J Am Acad Dermatol 2012;66(4):AB11.

66. Rotunda AM, Ablon G, Kolondey MS. Lipomas treated with subcutaneous deoxycholate injections. J Am Acad Dermatol 2005;53(6):973–8.

67. Kybella KPI. Deoxycholic acid) injection prescribing information. Westlake Village (CA): Kybella. 73179US10; 2018.

68. Deeks ED. Deoxycholic acid: a review in submental fat contouring. Am J Clin Dermatol 2016;17(6): 701–7.

69. Alacarini Farina GA, Cherubini K, Zancanaro de Figueiredo MA. Salum FG Deoxycholic acid in the submental fat reduction: a review of properties, adverse effects, and complications. J Cosmet Dermatol 2020;19(10):2497–504.

70. Souyoul S, Gioe O, Emerson A, et al. Alopecia after injection of ATX-101 for reduction of submental fat. JAAD Case Rep 2017;3(3):250–2.

71. Sebaratnam DF, Wond XL, Kim L, et al. Alopecia following deoxycholic acid treatment for submental adiposity. JAMA Facial Plast Surg 2019;21(6):571–2.

72. McKay C, Price C, Pruett L. Vascular injury after deoxycholic acid injection. Dermatol surg 2019;45(2): 306–9.

73. Lindgren AL, Welsh KM. Inadvertent intra-arterial injection of deoxycholic acid: a case report and proposed protocol for treatment. J Cosmet Dermatol 2020;19(7):1614–8.

74. Bernstein EF, Bloom JD. Safety and efficacy of bilateral submental cryolipolysis with quantified 3-dimensional imaging of fat reduction and skin tightening. JAMA Facial Plast Surg 2017;19(5):350–7.

75. Kilmer SL, Burns J A, elickson BD. Safety and efficacy of cryolipolysis for non-invasive reduction of submental fat. Lasers Surg Med 2016;48(1):3–13.

76. American Society of Plastic Surgeons (ASPS) 2020 ASPS National Clearinghouse of Plastic Surgery Procedural Statistics.

77. American Society of Plastic Surgeons (ASPS) 2018 ASPS National Clearinghouse of Plastic Surgery Procedural Statistics.

Noninvasive Hair Rejuvenation

Jordan Sand, MD[b], Scott Walen, MD[a],*

KEYWORDS

- Androgenetic alopecia • Hair rejuvenation • Medical therapy • Platelet-rich plasma

KEY POINTS

- There are several available noninvasive treatment options for androgenetic alopecia.
- Only 3 treatments are currently approved by Food and Drug Administration: minoxidil, finasteride, and low-light laser therapy.
- Many other treatment options are being used successfully in an off-label fashion, including platelet-rich plasma, microneedling, and topical finasteride.

BACKGROUND

Historically, hair thinning has been associated with the loss of youth, vitality, strength, and sexual attraction. Hair loss can reduce self-esteem, impair the quality of life, and negatively affect other's perceptions of the balding patient.[1] Androgenetic alopecia (AGA) is the most common hair loss disorder in both men and women. In general, AGA can start at a relatively early age, with 30% of men experiencing male pattern hair loss (MPHL) by age 30 years, 50% by age 50 years, and 80% by age 70 years.[2] Women are affected, but to a different degree, and through potentially different pathophysiologic pathways. Female pattern hair loss (FPHL) affects 3% to 12% of Caucasian women by age 30 years and 14% to 28% by age 60 years.[3] AGA can affect all ages, sexes, and ethnicities, but we know that both the incidence and severity of AGA increase with age in all groups and that the incidence of AGA is lower in Chinese, Japanese, and African men when compared with Caucasian men.[4]

HAIR PHYSIOLOGY

The hair cycle involves 4 distinct phases: anagen, catagen, telogen, and exogen (**Fig. 1**).

Approximately 50 to 100 hairs enter the exogen phase each day, shed, and then the anagen phase begins again with growth of a new hair follicle. In AGA, the ratio of hair in anagen phase to telogen phase decreases with each successive hair cycle. As a result, more hair is in telogen phase, which delays the cycle resuming the anagen phase. Each phase of the cycle contains specific events that often prepare the hair follicle to enter the subsequent phase (**Table 1**).

MPHL occurs in a predictable pattern, starting at the bitemporal region along the anterior hair line. With time the vertex and then the midfrontal regions of the scalp are involved; however, the occipital region is typically not involved to a significant degree. The classic progression of MPHL from bitemporal and vertex thinning, with a sparing of the temporal and occipital hair, is described in 7-point grading system originated by Norwood, which is used by practitioners all over the world (**Fig. 2**).[5] In contrast, FPHL is considered a different entity, with a different presentation. Typically, FPHL presents with a more diffuse, central thinning over the midfrontal scalp, with preservation of the bitemporal anterior hairline, and vertex regions. This pattern was originally described by Ludwig, and the resulting classification scale is used for FPHL (**Fig. 3**).[6]

[a] Division of Facial Plastic and Reconstructive Surgery, Department of Otolaryngology-Head and Neck Surgery, The Pennsylvania State University, College of Medicine, 500 University Drive H-091, Hershey, PA 17033, USA;
[b] Spokane Center for Facial Plastic Surgery, 217 W. Cataldo Avenue, Spokane, WA 99201, USA
* Corresponding author.
E-mail address: swalen1@pennstatehealth.psu.edu

Facial Plast Surg Clin N Am 30 (2022) 419–431
https://doi.org/10.1016/j.fsc.2022.03.015
1064-7406/22/© 2022 Elsevier Inc. All rights reserved.

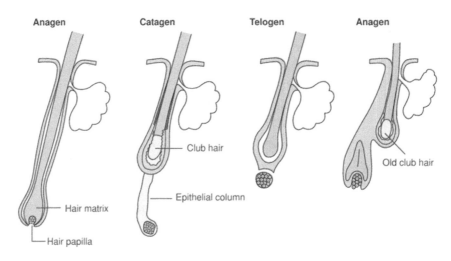

Anagen   Catagen   Telogen   Anagen

Club hair

Old club hair

Epithelial column

Hair matrix

Hair papilla

Diagrammatic representation of the scalp hair cycle

Published in Expert Reviews in Molecular Medicine by Cambridge University Press (2002)

Fig. 1. Stages of the hair cycle. (*Reproduced from* Sinclair R. Male pattern androgenetic alopecia BMJ 1998; 317 :865 doi:10.1136/bmj.317.7162.865. © 1998, with permission from BMJ Publishing Group Ltd.)

THERAPEUTIC OPTIONS
First-Line Treatments

Minoxidil

Minoxidil was incidentally found to work as a powerful vasodilator, which leads to its development as an antihypertensive drug. The favored theory is that the vasodilation action of minoxidil increases blood supply to the scalp (**Fig. 4B**).[7] Initial trials were performed that showed moderate to significant hair growth in ~40% of the patients enrolled.[8] The 2% formulation received approval from Food and Drug Administration (FDA) for treatment of AGA in male and female patients in 1998 and 2001, respectively. The 5% topical foam preparation was FDA approved for men in 2006, and the 5% solution was also FDA approved for men in 2007.[9] Currently, the 5% foam or solution is not FDA approved for use in women, but off-label use is common.[10]

There have been several randomized control trials (RCTs) assessing both 2% versus 5% minoxidil against each other and against placebo. Minoxidil 2% has been shown to be effective in preventing progression of AGA and improving AGA in the frontotemporal and vertex areas in men.[11] Furthermore, 5% minoxidil solution or foam has been shown to be more effective than the 2% solution. One study comparing the 2% and 5% solution of minoxidil found a 60% increase in cosmetic results in the 5% group compared with 40% in the 2% group.[12]

Although men have been more studied than women for alopecia, there are several high-quality studies showing promise in treating FPHL. Minoxidil 2% solution twice daily has been shown to prevent progression and improve AGA in female patients. The efficacy of 5% minoxidil solution or foam applied once daily was no different

Table 1
Stages of the hair cycle

	Stage	Length	% of Hair	Processes
Anagen	Active growth	2–6 y	90	Dermal papilla increase size GF's secreted HF grows 1 cm/28 d
Catagen	Transition phase	2–4 wk	1–2	Matrix degenerates HF cut off from blood supply At the end, 1/6 of original length
Telogen	Resting phase	3–5 mo	10	Fully keratinized, "club hair" Once keratinized, shed (50–100/d) Signals begin move to anagen

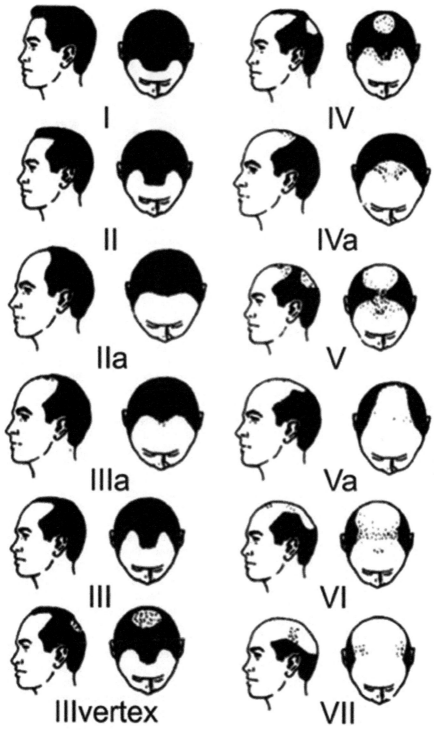

I
II
IIa
IIIa
III
IIIvertex

IV
IVa
V
Va
VI
VII

Fig. 2. Norwood-Hamilton staging for MPHL. (Francisco Jimenez, Majid Alam, James E. Vogel, Marc Avram, Hair transplantation: Basic overview, Journal of the American Academy of Dermatology, 85(4), 2021, 803-814, https://doi.org/10.1016/j.jaad.2021.03.124.)

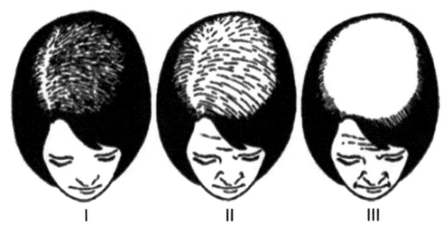

Fig. 3. Ludwig staging for FPHL. (LUDWIG, E. (1977), Classification of the types of androgenetic alopecia (common baldness) occurring in the female sex. British Journal of Dermatology, 97: 247-254. https://doi.org/10.1111/j.1365-2133.1977.tb15179.x.)

when compared with the 2% minoxidil applied twice daily.[13]

Minoxidil treatment should be used for 6 months before assessing the final results. Patients should be warned that there could be a transient period of hair shedding at the 2-month mark. The minoxidil should be spread onto the scalp and left in place for approximately 4 hours. Patients should also be advised that drug interruption will cause acute hair shedding after 3 to 4 months but that hair shedding involves only the hairs that were going to be lost before treatment.[14]

Finasteride

Finasteride is an oral medication that has been FDA approved at a dose of 1 mg daily for use in men with AGA since 1997. The mechanism of action is through the selectively inhibition of type II 5-alpha reductase (AR), found in hair follicles and the prostate, which produces dihydrotestosterone (DHT) from testosterone (Fig. 4A); this results in a reduced level of DHT in both the serum and scalp, but increases the level of testosterone in the scalp.[15] Through the blocking of DHT, finasteride restores the proper length of the anagen phase, which results in an increased growth rate and hair width.[16]

Finasteride at a dose of 1 mg daily has been shown to increase the hair count, physician-assessed hair coverage, and hair mass compared with placebo.[17,18] A systematic review of the efficacy of finasteride in men with male pattern hair loss found that 5.6 patients need to be treated short term, and 3.4 patients need to be treated long term, for one patient to perceive an improvement. There was a 20% absolute increase in patient-perceived improvement in the short term and a 30% absolute increase in the long term. Longer treatment with finasteride promotes

greater therapeutic success.[19] Similar to minoxidil, response to finasteride varies, and hair regrowth can be lost after the medication is discontinued.

In contrast, finasteride is not FDA approved for the treatment of FPHL. A study looking at a small population of Asian women showed improvements in hair density, width, and scalp appearance after 1 year of finasteride use.[20] A double-blind, placebo-controlled, randomized multicenter trial found finasteride, 1 mg, to be ineffective in postmenopausal women with female pattern hair loss at 12 months.[21,22] The results of finasteride overall show similar promise in FPHL, but they are on a small population and inconsistent. Further studies will be required to assess ideal dosage and efficacy of finasteride for FPHL.

The recommended dose of finasteride of 1 mg/d and the result should be assessed at 6 to 12 months. Side effects from finasteride include decreased libido, erectile dysfunction, gynecomastia, and depression. Postfinasteride syndrome is a constellation of sexual, somatic, and psychological disorders that persist after cessation of treatment, independent of age, dosage, or indication.[23] The side effects of finasteride in women have been studied less than in men, but there have been reports of decreased libido, dry skin, mild acne, headache, dizziness, irregular menses, hypertrichosis, and changes in liver enzymes.[24] Because of its antiandrogenic effects, pregnant women are advised against coming into physical contact with finasteride. Doing so may inhibit the proper sexual development of male fetuses or induce genital abnormalities.[25]

Laser- and light-based therapy

Low-level laser therapy (LLLT) is one of the few FDA-cleared devices used for treatment of

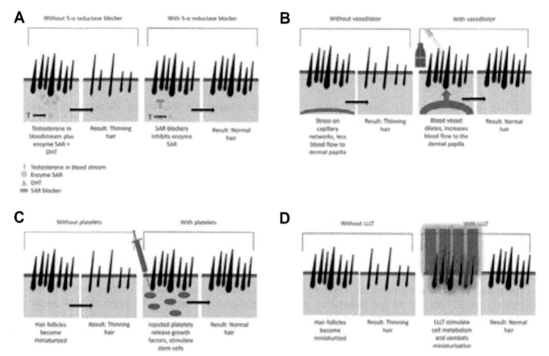

Fig. 4. (*A*) Working hypothesis of antiandrogens in AGA. (*B*) Working hypothesis of vasodilator in AGA. (*C*) Working hypothesis of PRP in AGA. (*D*) Working hypothesis of LLLT in AGA. (*From* Gupta AK, Mays RR, Dotzert MS, Versteeg SG, Shear NH, Piguet V. Efficacy of non-surgical treatments for androgenetic alopecia: a systematic review and network meta-analysis. J Eur Acad Dermatol Venereol. 2018 Dec;32(12):2112-2125; with permission.)

alopecia. LLLT works by a process called photo-biomodulation, where the laser stimulates a specific biological process in the target tissue. LLLT wavelengths typically fall between 500 and 1100 nm with a power density between 5 and 500 mW. The precise mechanism of action is not known, but there are several postulations. LLLT generates oxygen radicals and antioxidants, which increase keratinocyte and fibroblast mitosis. Another theory involves the generation of adenosine triphosphate through inhibiting nitric oxide, which can increase metabolism and abate apoptosis, which causes new hair growth.[26] A final thought is that the LLLT decreases inflammation through decreased prostaglandin E-2, and increasing antiinflammatory cytokines, thereby activating hair growth. These effects are thought to prolong the anagen phase of the hair cycle, stimulate hair follicles that are into the telogen phase to reenter the anagen phase, and inhibit the early entry into the catagen phase (**Fig. 4**D).[27]

A 2020 literature review by Egger and colleagues found 10 RCTs with similar treatment settings, duration, and objective endpoints. Eight of the studies compared LLLT technology with sham devices, and all 8 found a statistically significant increase in hair diameter or density. Five of the studies analyzed included patient satisfaction

metrics; in most cases, the treatment group showed a more favorable assessment than the control group. They concluded that these devices work well in men and women with AGA, with minimal adverse effects reported.[28] Recently, Gentile performed a systematic review of LLLT for both MPHL and FPHL. All 7 RCTs analyzed showed an improvement in hair count and density, in both men and women, in mild to moderate AGA.[29]

When looking at the totality of clinical trials, reported adverse effects are minimal. In a 2018 review, out of 13 studies, 5 showed adverse side effects including acne, mild paresthesia, urticaria, headache/scalp tenderness, and pruritis in a small fraction of patients. No adverse effects required disruption or discontinuation of treatment, and most resolved within 2 weeks.[30] Overall, LLLT is clearly an important treatment modality, as there are several FDA-cleared devices including the Hair-Max Lasercomb, iGrow, Theradome, and the Capillus laser cap, all using low-level laser technology in an effort to treat patients with hair loss (**Fig. 5**).

Second-Line Treatments

Microneedling
Microneedling (MN) is a minimally invasive procedure that uses fine needles to puncture the outer

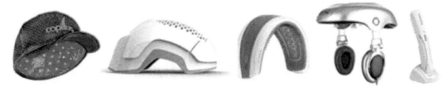

Fig. 5. Examples of various LLLT devices (Left to Right: Capillus Laser Cap, Theradome, HairMax Laser Band 82, iGrow Laser Helmet, and HairMax Laser Comb).

surface of the skin, the stratum corneum. Previous to its use in alopecia, it has been used in skin rejuvenation, scar treatments, acne treatment, burns, melasma, and keloids.[31] Typically, MN is performed by using a roller or a needle pen over the scalp that contain needles with various depths of penetration between 0.8 and 2.5 mm. The mechanism of action is thought to be partially due to the local trauma from the needles that stimulate the tissue's own growth factors.[32]

Dhurat and colleagues randomized 100 patients comparing weekly MN treatment plus twice-daily minoxidil 5% with minoxidil alone. The MN group had a significantly greater hair count at 12 weeks.[33] Generally, MN is thought to be tolerated well by patients with the adverse effects including bleeding, pain, redness, and scalp irritation. From the literature, it seems that MN is being combined with other first-line treatments including minoxidil and platelet-rich plasma (PRP).[34] MN is thought to increase the penetration of topical therapies, allowing a greater absorption of large molecules[32]; this is a well-tolerated procedure with only mild side effects such as itching, redness, and folliculitis reported.[35]

Platelet-rich plasma

PRP is a relatively new treatment that has been used in several surgical fields including cardiac surgery, dentistry, ophthalmology, orthopedics, and plastic surgery. Within plastic surgery, PRP is used to improve healing, augment tissue, promote stem cell growth, and as an off-label treatment of AGA (**Fig. 4**C). PRP is an autogenously harvested serum that is processed to concentrate various growth factors and platelets.[36] The growth factors contained in PRP include platelet-derived growth factor, transforming growth factor β, vascular endothelial growth factor, epidermal growth factor, and insulinlike growth factor. These factors are known to be mitogenic to several cell types including monocytes, fibroblasts, stem cells, endothelial cells, and keratinocytes. They have also been shown to increase angiogenesis, increase collagen production, and allow increased cellular permeability (see **Table 1**).[37]

In 2006, Uebel and colleagues were the first to show the potentially positive effects of PRP after hair follicles used for hair transplantation were treated with PRP and showed increased growth and density.[38] In 2016, Alves and colleagues published an RCT looking at 25 patients injected with PRP in one-half of the scalp and saline in the other. At 3- and 6-month intervals, there was an increase in mean anagen hairs, telogen hairs, hair density, and terminal hair density compared with baseline. They also found that mean total hair density, male sex, age less than 40 years, beginning of hair loss at an age greater than 25 years, positive family history, and greater than 10 years of AGA could predict a potential better outcome (**Fig. 6**).[39]

When looking at the effect in women, Puig published an RCT where 26 women were injected with either PRP or saline one time. At 26 weeks, there was no statistical difference in hair count or hair mass, but more subjects in the PRP-treated group reported improvement in hair loss, rate of hair loss, an increase in thickness, and heavier/coarser hair.[40] Gentile performed a systematic review in 2020 looking at 12 trials showing that 84% showed a positive effect of PRP on AGA, 50% of the studies showed a statistically significant improvement of objective measures, and 34% reported an improvement in hair thickness and density. Only 9% (1 study) of the studies reported that PRP was not effective in treating AGA.[41]

One drawback of PRP is the lack of consensus on the exact concentration, the utility of activators, dosing parameters, depth of injection, or frequency of sessions. In general, the studies that showed that PRP had a positive effect on AGA had at least 3 treatments, spaced 1 month apart, and further maintenance treatments yearly. Typically, the PRP is injected at the dermal/subdermal junction, one inch apart, and evenly distributed around the areas of hair loss.[42] Transient pain and erythema are the most common side effects of PRP injections, with no major adverse effects reported in the literature.[43]

Dutasteride

Dutasteride, a potent type I and type II 5-AR inhibitor, is used to treat benign prostatic hyperplasia but is also prescribed as an off-label treatment of pattern hair loss, more specifically, in patients who have not responded to finasteride. One RCT

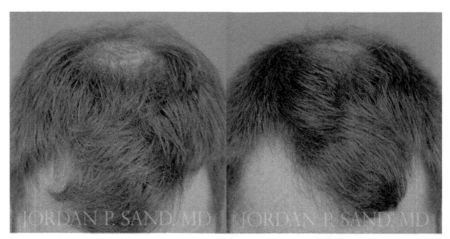

Fig. 6. A 47-year-old man with AGA before (left) and 6 months after 3 monthly PRP (right) treatments.

in 416 men with male pattern hair loss demonstrated that dutasteride, 2.5 mg, was superior to finasteride, 5 mg, in terms of increasing hair count over 24 weeks.[44] Zhou and colleagues performed a meta-analysis looking at the safety and efficacy of dutasteride against finasteride in treating AGA over a 24-week cycle. The metanalysis contained 3 RCTs and showed that dutasteride showed an improvement in total hair count, physician assessment of global photographs, and subject assessment. In addition, there was no significant difference in patient safety, with similar rates of altered libido, erectile dysfunction, and ejaculation disorders.[45]

Jung and colleagues took 31 patients with no clinical response to finasteride and placed them on dutasteride; 77.4% of these patients showed an improvement on dutasteride.[46] Finally, Shanshanwal and Dhurat performed a comparative, randomized, evaluator-blinded study in 90 male patients, which showed an increase in total hair count by 5-fold in the dutasteride group over finasteride. Interestingly, they also noted an increase in thin hair count, where they used a surrogate for reversal of hair follicle miniaturization. The finasteride group showed no increase in thin hair count.[47] There is no significant difference in adverse effects between dutasteride, 0.5 mg daily, and finasteride, 1 mg daily.[44] Similar to finasteride, caution should be given to starting women of child-bearing age on dutasteride.

Antiandrogens

Antiandrogen therapy with spironolactone, cyproterone acetate (CA), or flutamide are used for treatment of FPHL, despite limited evidence.[9] CA blocks androgen receptors and decreases luteinizing hormone/follicle stimulating hormone release, which decreases testosterone. One study found that CA/

ethinyl estradiol (2 mg/0.035 mg) taken daily in 35 women resulted in both a cessation of hair loss in 83% of subjects and also hair regrowth in 77%.[48] Treatment with CA has been shown to improve hair growth in patients with FPHL, with both normal and high androgen levels.[49]

Spironolactone is a potassium-sparing diuretic, which reduces testosterone levels and competitively blocks androgen receptors in target tissues.[48] The role of spironolactone has been studied and found to be potentially effective in FPHL, both on its own and combined with minoxidil.[50,51] The starting dose is typically between 50 and 200 mg daily, and response should only be assessed after 6 months. Side effects of antiandrogens can include postural hypotension, electrolyte disturbances (hyperkalemia with spironolactone), menstrual irregularities, fatigue, urticaria, and breast tenderness.[52] Despite some initial promise, neither oral or topical antiandrogens are recommended for hair loss except for cyproterone acetate in hyperandrogenic women.[9] Oral contraception is recommended to prevent pregnancy in premenopausal women, as spironolactone can cause feminization of the male fetus.

Ketoconazole

Ketoconazole is an imidazole antifungal that is predominantly used in shampoo form for seborrheic dermatitis. It acts as an antiinflammatory and an androgen-receptor antagonist. Topical ketoconazole 2% shampoo may also have some efficacy in treatment of AGA; a small trial of 39 men with AGA showed an increase in hair density after 6 months of treatment.[53] Ketoconazole can also work as an adjunct when combined with finasteride to further decrease DHT levels.[54] A 2020 systematic review showed an increase in hair shaft

Table 2
Medical treatment options for androgenetic alopecia

Medication	Intended Population	Method of Administration	Mechanism of Action	Frequency/Duration	FDA Approval Status	Adverse Effects
Minoxidil[a]	M, F	Topical	Vasodilation, antiandrogenic, antiinflammatory	Daily >6 mo	Approved	• Hypertrichosis • Contact dermatitis
Finasteride[a]	M	Oral	5-α-reductase inhibitor	Daily >6 mo	Approved	• Sexual side effects • Mood disturbances
Dutasteride	M	Oral	5-α-reductase inhibitor	Daily >6 mo	Not approved, approved in other countries	• Sexual side effects • Mood disturbances
Spironolactone	F	Oral	Potassium-sparing diuretic	Daily >6 mo	Not approved for AGA	• Hyperkalemia • Sexual side effects • Feminization • Orthostatic hypotension
Oral minoxidil	M, F	Oral	Vasodilation, antiandrogenic, antiinflammatory	Daily >6 mo	Not approved for AGA	• Hypotension • Lower limb edema • Hypertrichosis
Topical finasteride	M, F	Topical	5-α-reductase inhibitor	Daily >6 mo	Not approved for AGA	• Systematic absorbtion with same sexual and mood problems as oral
Latanoprost	M, F	Topical	Prostaglandin analogue, prolongs anagen phase	Daily >6 mo	Not approved for AGA	• Erythematous reaction
Ketoconazole	M, F	Topical	Imidazole antifungal, antiinflammatory	Daily >6 mo	Not approved for AGA	• Itching, burning • Dry skin

[a] Authors' first-line treatment of AGA.

Table 3
Adjuvant procedures for androgenetic alopecia

Treatment	Mechanism	Protocol	FDA Approval Status	Adverse Effects
Low-level laser therapy	• Stimulation anagen • Activation dormant follicles • Increase ATP, GFs	• 3x per wk, 15–25 min • Every other day, 25–30 min • >6 mo	Approved	• Photosensitivity
Platelet-rich plasma (PRP)	• Differentiation of stem cells into hair follicles • Prolong anlagen phase • Prevent hair cells from apoptosis	• Monthly for 3 mo, maintenance treatment yearly[a] • 2/3 sessions at 3-mo interval	Not approved	• Pain, irritation at site • Bleeding
Scalp microneedling	• Release of PDGF • Activation of follicular stem cells • Inflammation to puncture site	• May combine with PRP • Alone, 1 session per wk for 12 wk	Not approved	• Pain, irritation at site • Bleeding • Telogen effluvium • Lymph node enlargement
Adipose tissue injections	• Improve vascularity and blood supply to scalp • Delivery of early induced PGDF, FGF, VEGF	• 1 session of injections	Not approved	• Pain, dermatitis • Recurrence of alopecia

Abbreviations: ATP, adenosine; FGF, fibroblast growth factor; GF, growth factors; PDGF, platelet-derived growth factor; VEGF, vascular endothelial growth factor.
[a] Authors' preferred PRP protocol.

diameter with ketoconazole use, in addition to improvements on clinical photographs and subjective evaluations of AGA.[55]

Prostaglandins

Prostaglandin (PG) levels are unregulated in AGA and could be of importance in discovering an effective treatment modality. Recent studies have shown a role for prostaglandins in hair growth. Latanoprost and bimatoprost, both PG-F2 analogues, have been shown to prolong the anagen phase and stimulate hair growth.[56] One RCT with 16 male patients showed improvement in hair density using topical latanoprost 0.1%.[57] PG-E2 analogues have been shown to protect hair loss in radiated mice.[58] Elevated PG-D2 levels, in contrast, are known to increase miniaturization and inhibit hair growth.[59] Adverse effects tend to only be located at the treatment site and include erythema and folliculitis.[57]

Topical finasteride

Recently, topical finasteride has been studied and shown to have promise in both MPHL and FPHL.[60] Topical finasteride is used at a far lower dose than the oral version, which minimizes potential side effects, and allows use in women of reproductive age. One study looked at 52 men and premenopausal women treated with 0.005% topical finasteride applied twice daily for 16 months. There was a significant reduction in hair loss starting at the sixth month of treatment, which extended to the end of the study.[61] Postmenopausal women were also studied in an RCT looking at 3% minoxidil alone versus 3% minoxidil and 0.25% finasteride. There was an increase in hair diameter at week 24, and clinical improvements were seen in 90% of the study group. The side-effect profile includes itching, irritation, and lowered serum DHT in women.[62]

Oral minoxidil

Oral minoxidil works through a similar mechanism as the topical form. It has been studied at a dose of 0.25 mg alone and in combination with spironolactone in FPHL.[52] The current evidence does show efficacy of 5 mg daily for MPHL and 0.25 mg daily with 25 mg spironolactone for FPHL.[63] At higher doses (5 mg and higher), oral minoxidil may cause pedal edema, postural hypotension, and electrocardiogram abnormalities.[52]

SUMMARY

Hair loss affects both men and women and may start at an early age. Three FDA-approved treatments for AGA exist: minoxidil, finasteride, and LLLT (numerous devices). There are several other potential promising non–FDA-approved treatments including PRP injections ± microneedling, antiandrogens, prostaglandin analogues, and adipose injections (Tables 2 and 3). Despite the many options, treatments typically take 6 to 12 months before a clinically objective result may occur, and once the treatment starts, it must continue indefinitely to sustain the results.

CLINICS CARE POINTS

- MPHL and FPHL can cause distress to patients but the pathology may be different, in addition to, the potential side effects of treatment.
- Both minoxidil and finasteride are commonly prescribed and have positive results in the treatment of AGA.
- LLLT also show promising results and can be used as a solo modality and in combination with other treatments for AGA.
- PRP treatments are showing positive results in both MPHL and FPHL, but more rigorous studies need to be performed.
- Aside from hair transplantation, many of the current therapies for AGA must be continued on an ongoing basis; therefore compliance is of utmost importance.

DISCLOSURE

The authors have nothing to disclose.

REFERENCES

1. Cash TF. The psychological effects of androgenetic alopecia in men. J Am Acad Dermatol 1992;26(6): 926–31.
2. Cash TF, Price VH, Savin RC. Psychological effects of androgenetic alopecia on women: comparisons with balding men and with female control subjects. J Am Acad Dermatol 1993;29(4):568–75.
3. Ellis JA, Sinclair R, Harrap SB. Androgenetic alopecia: pathogenesis and potential for therapy. Expert Rev Mol Med 2002;4(22):1–11.
4. Severi G, Sinclair R, Hopper JL, et al. Androgenetic alopecia in men aged 40-69 years: prevalence and risk factors. Br J Dermatol 2003;149(6):1207–13.
5. Norwood OT. Male pattern baldness: classification and incidence. South Med J 1975;68(11):1359–65.
6. Ludwig E. Classification of the types of androgenetic alopecia (common baldness) occurring in the female sex. Br J Dermatol 1977;97(3):247–54.

7. Wester RC, Maibach HI, Guy RH, et al. Minoxidil stimulates cutaneous blood flow in human balding scalps: pharmacodynamics measured by laser Doppler velocimetry and photopulse plethysmography. J Invest Dermatol 1984;82:515–7.

8. Devine BL, Fife R, Trust PM. Minoxidil for severe hypertension after failure of other hypotensive drugs. Br Med J 1977;ii:667.

9. Blumeyer A, Tosti A, Messenger A, et al. European Dermatology Forum (EDF). Evidence-based (S3) guideline for the treatment of androgenetic alopecia in women and in men. J Dtsch Dermatol Ges 2011; 9(Suppl 6):S1–57.

10. Alves R, Grimalt R. Androgenetic alopecia in adolescents. In: Oranje AP, Al-Mutairi N, Shwayder T, editors. Practical pediatric dermatology. controversies in diagnosis and treatment. Switzerland: Springer; 2016. p. 187–96.

11. Kanti V, Hillmann K, Kottner J, et al. Effect of minoxidil topical foam on frontotemporal and vertex androgenetic alopecia in men: a 104-week open-label clinical trial. J Eur Acad Dermatol Venereol 2016; 30(7):1183–9.

12. Olsen EA, Dunlap FE, Funicella T, et al. A randomized clinical trial of 5% topical minoxidil versus 2% topical minoxidil and placebo in the treatment of androgenetic alopecia in men. J Am Acad Dermatol 2002;47(3):377–85.

13. Kanti V, Messenger A, Dobos G, et al. Evidence-based(S3) guideline for the treatment of androgenetic alopecia in women and in men – short version. J Eur Acad Dermatol Venereol 2018;32(1):11–22.

14. Rietschel RL, Duncan SH. Safety and efficacy of topical minoxidil in the management of androgenetic alopecia. J Am Acad Dermatol 1987;16(3 Pt 2):677–85.

15. Rhodes L, Harper J, Uno H, et al. The effects of finasteride (Proscar) on hair growth, hair cycle stage, and serum testosterone and dihydrotestosterone in adult male and female stumptail macaques (Macaca arctoides). J Clin Endocrinol Metab 1994;79:991–6.

16. Whiting DA, Waldstreicher J, Sanchez M, et al. Measuring reversal of hair miniaturization in androgenetic alopecia by follicular counts in horizontal sections of serial scalp biopsies: results of finasteride 1 mg treatment of men and postmenopausal women. J Investig Dermatol Symp Proc 1999;4(3): 282–4.

17. Drake L, Hordinsky M, Fiedler V, et al. The effects of finasteride on scalp skin and serum androgen levels in men with androgenetic alopecia. J Amacad Dermatol 1999;41(4):550–4.

18. Stough DB, Rao NA, Kaufman KD, et al. Finasteride improves male pattern hair loss in a randomized study in identical twins. Eur J Dermatol 2002;12(1): 32–7.

19. Mella JM, Perret MC, Manzotti M, et al. Efficacy and safety of finasteride therapy for androgenetic alopecia: a systematic review. Arch Dermatol 2010; 146(10):1141–50.

20. Yeon JH, Jung JY, Choi JW, et al. 5 mg/day finasteride treatment for normoandrogenic Asian women with female pattern hair loss. J Eur Acad Dermatol Venereol 2011;25(2):211–4.

21. Price VH, Roberts JL, Hordinsky M, et al. Lack of efficacy of finasteride in postmenopausal women with androgenetic alopecia. J Am Acad Dermatol 2000; 43(5, pt 1):768–76.

22. McClellan KJ, Finasteride MA. A review of its use in male pattern hair loss. Drugs 1999;57:111–26.

23. Trüeb RM, Régnier A, Dutra Rezende H, et al. Post-Finasteride Syndrome: An Induced Delusional Disorder with the Potential of a Mass Psychogenic Illness? Skin Appendage Disord 2019; 5:320–6.

24. Oliveira-Soares R, Silva JM, Correia MP, et al. Finasteride 5 mg/day treatment of patterned hair loss in normo-androgenetic postmenopausal women. Int J Trichol 2013;5:22–5.

25. Hu AC, Chapman LW, Mesinkovska NA. The efficacy and use of finasteride in women: a systematic review. Int J Dermatol 2019;58:759–76.

26. Farivar S, Malekshahabi T, Shiari R. Biological effects of low level laser therapy. J Laser Med Sci 2014;5:58–62.

27. Sakurai Y, Yamaguchi M, Abiko Y. Inhibitory effect of low-level laser irradiation on LPS-stimulated prostaglandin E2 production and cyclooxygenase-2 in human gingival fibroblasts. Eur J Oral Sci 2000;108: 29–34.

28. Egger A, Resnik S R, Aickara D, et al. Examining the safety and efficacy of low-level laser therapy for male and female pattern hair loss: a review of the literature. Skin Appendage Disord 2020;6:259–67.

29. Gentile Pietro, Garcovich Simone. The Effectiveness of Low-Level Light/Laser Therapy on Hair Loss. Facial Plast Surg Aesthet Med 2021. https://doi.org/10.1089/fpsam.2021.0151.

30. Darwin E, Heyes A, Hirt PA, et al. Low-level laser therapy for the treatment of androgenic alopecia: a review. Lasers Med Sci 2018;33(2):425–34.

31. Hou A, Cohen B, Haimovic A, et al. Microneedling: a comprehensive review. Dermatol Surg 2017;43: 321–39.

32. Singh A, Yadav S. Microneedling: advances and widening horizons. Indian Dermatol Online J 2016; 7:244–54.

33. Dhurat R, Sukesh M, Avhad G, et al. A randomized evaluator blinded study of effect of microneedling in androgenetic alopecia: a pilot study. Int J Trichol 2013;5:6–11.

34. Kumar MK, Inamadar AC, Palit A. A randomized controlled single-observer blinded study to determine the efficacy of topical minoxidil plus microneedling versus topical minoxidil alone in the treatment

of androgenetic alopecia. J Cutan Aesthet Surg 2018;11:211–6.

35. Neerja P. A study on the efficacy of microneedling with minoxidil solution versus microneedling with hair multivitamin solution for the treatment of androgenetic alopecia. Int J Dermatol Clin Res 2020;6(1): 010–2.

36. Kang RS, Lee MK, Seth R, et al. Platelet-rich plasma in cosmetic surgery. Int J Otorhinolaryngol Clin 2013;5(01):24–8.

37. Sclafani AP, Romo T III, Ukrainsky G, et al. Modulation of wound response and soft tissue ingrowth in synthetic and allogeneic implants with platelet concentrate. Arch Facial Plast Surg 2005;7(03): 163–9.

38. Uebel CO, da Silva JB, Cantarelli D, et al. The role of platelet plasma growth factors in male pattern baldness surgery. Plast Reconstr Surg 2006;118: 1458–67.

39. Alves R, Grimalt R. Randomized placebo-controlled, double-blind,half-head study to assess the efficacy of platelet-rich plasma on the treatment of androgenetic alopecia. Dermatol Surg 2016;42(04):491–7.

40. Puig CJ, Reese R, PetersM. Double- blind, placebo-controlled pilot study on the use of platelet-rich plasma in women with female androgenetic alopecia. Dermatol Surg 2016;42(11):1243–7.

41. Gentile P, Garcovich S. Systematic Review of Platelet-Rich Plasma Use in Androgenetic Alopecia Compared with Minoxidil, Finasteride, and Adult Stem Cell-Based Therapy. Int J Mol Sci 2020;21(8): 2702.

42. Gupta AK, Versteeg SG, Rapaport J, et al. The efficacy of platelet-rich plasma in the field of hair restoration and facial aesthetics-A systematic review and meta-analysis. J Cutan Med Surg 2019;23(2): 185–203.

43. Jha AK, Vinay K, Zeeshan M, et al. Platelet-rich plasma and microneedling improves hair growth in patients of androgenetic alopecia when used as an adjuvant to minoxidil. J Cosmet Dermatol 2019; 18:1330–5.

44. Olsen EA, Hordinsky M, Whiting D, et al. The importance of dual 5alpha-reductase inhibition in the treatment of male pattern hair loss: Results of a randomized placebo-controlled study of dutasteride versus finasteride. J Am Acad Dermatol 2006;55: 1014–23.

45. Zhou Z, Song S, Gao Z, et al. The efficacy and safety of dutasteride compared with finasteride in treating men with androgenetic alopecia: a systematic review and meta-analysis. Clin Interv Aging 2019;14: 399–406.

46. Jung JY, Yeon JH, Choi JW, et al. Effect of dutasteride 0.5 mg/d in men with androgenetic alopecia recalcitrant to finasteride. Int J Dermatol 2014; 53(11):1351–7.

47. Shanshanwal SJ, Dhurat RS. Superiority of dutasteride over finasteride in hair regrowth and reversal of miniaturization in men with androgenetic alopecia: a randomized controlled open-label, evaluator-blinded study. Indian J Dermatol Venereol Leprol 2017;83(1):47–54.

48. Coneac A, Muresan A, Orasan MS. Antiandrogenic therapy with ciproterone acetate in female patients who suffer from both androgenetic alopecia and acne vulgaris. Clujul Med 2014;87(4): 226–34.

49. Karrer-Voegeli S, Rey F, Reymond MJ, et al. Androgen dependence of hirsutism, acne and alopecia in women: a prospective analysis of 228 patients investigated for hyperandrogenism. Medicine(Baltimore) 2009;88(1):32–45.

50. Sinclair R, Wewerinke M, Jolley D. Treatment of female pattern hair loss with oral antiandrogens. Br J Dermatol 2005;152:466–73.

51. Brough KR, Torgerson RR. Hormonal therapy in female pattern hair loss. Int J Womens Dermatol 2017;3:53–7.

52. Sinclair RD. Female pattern hair loss: a pilot study investigating combination therapy with low-dose oral minoxidil and spironolactone. Int J Dermatol 2018;57:104–9.

53. Piérard-Franchimont C, De Doncker P, Cauwenbergh G, et al. Ketoconazole shampoo: effect of long-term use in androgenic alopecia. Dermatology 1998;196:474–7.

54. Hugo Perez BS. Ketocazole as an adjunct to finasteride in the treatment of androgenetic alopecia in men. Med Hypotheses 2004;62(1):112–5.

55. Fields JR, Vonu PM, Monir RL, et al. Topical ketoconazole for the treatment of androgenetic alopecia: a systematic review. Dermatol Ther 2020;33(1): e13202.

56. Valente Duarte De Sousa IC, Tosti A. New investigational drugs for androgenetic alopecia. Expert Opin Investig Drugs 2013;22:573–89.

57. Blume-Peytavi U, Lönnfors S, Hillmann K, et al. A randomized double-blind placebo-controlled pilot study to assess the efficacy of a 24-week topical treatment by latanoprost 0.1% on hair growth and pigmentation in healthy volunteers with androgenetic alopecia. J Am Acad Dermatol 2012;66(5): 794–800.

58. Geng L, Hanson WR, Malkinson FD. Topical or systemic 16,16 Dm prostaglandin E2 or WR-2721 (WR-1065) protects mice from alopecia after fractionated irradiation. Int J Radiat Biol 1992;61: 533–7.

59. Nieves A, Garza LA. Does prostaglandin D2 hold the cure to male pattern baldness? Exp Dermatol 2014; 23(4):224–7.

60. Suchonwanit P, Srisuwanwattana P, Chalermroj N, et al. A randomized, double-blind controlled study

of the efficacy and safety of topical solution of 0.25% finasteride admixed with 3% minoxidil vs. 3% minoxidil solution in the treatment of male androgenetic alopecia. J Eur Acad Dermatol Venereol 2018;32: 2257–63.

61. Mazzarella GF, Loconsole GF, Cammisa GA, et al. Topical finasteride in the treatment of androgenic alopecia. Preliminary evaluations after a 16-month therapy course. J Dermatolog Treat 1997;8: 189–92.

62. Suchonwanit P, Iamsumang W, Rojhirunsakool S. Efficacy of topical combination of 0.25% finasteride and 3% minoxidil versus 3% minoxidil solution in female pattern hair loss: a randomized, double-blind, controlled study. Am J Clin Dermatol 2019;20: 147–53.

63. Lueangarun S, Panchapreteep R, Tempark T, et al. Efficacy and safety of oral minoxidil 5 mg daily during 24-week treatment in male androgenetic alopecia. J Am Acad Dermatol 2015;72:AB113.

Moving?

Make sure your subscription moves with you!

To notify us of your new address, find your **Clinics Account Number** (located on your mailing label above your name), and contact customer service at:

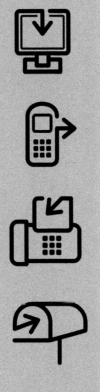

Email: **journalscustomerservice-usa@elsevier.com**

800-654-2452 (subscribers in the U.S. & Canada)
314-447-8871 (subscribers outside of the U.S. & Canada)

Fax number: **314-447-8029**

Elsevier Health Sciences Division
Subscription Customer Service
3251 Riverport Lane
Maryland Heights, MO 63043

*To ensure uninterrupted delivery of your subscription, please notify us at least 4 weeks in advance of move.

9780323850056